making
transparent
SOAP

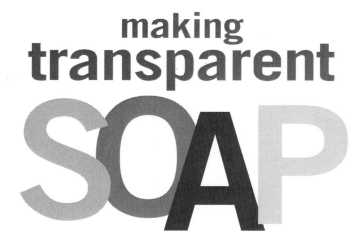

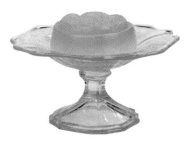

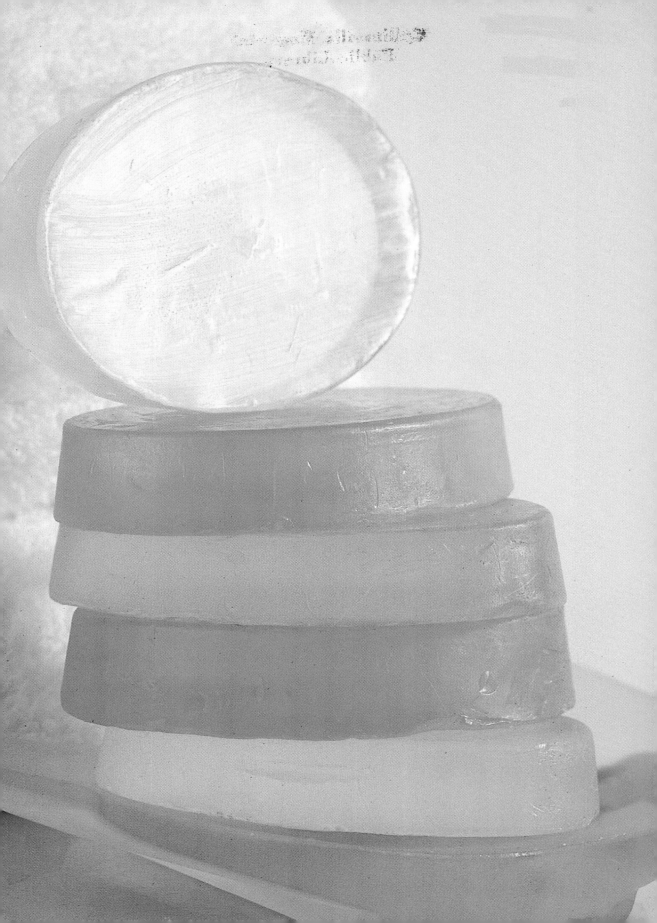

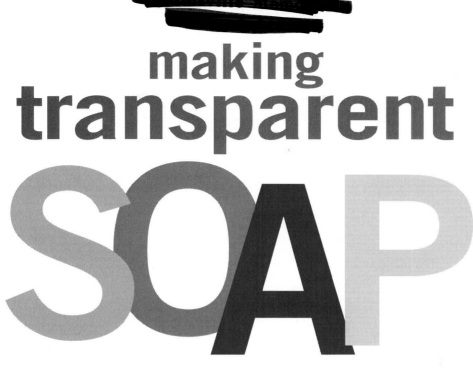

making
transparent
SOAP

the art of
crafting, molding,
scenting & coloring

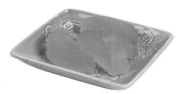

catherine failor

STOREY
BOOKS

Schoolhouse Road
Pownal, Vermont 05261

The mission of Storey Communications is to serve our customers by publishing practical information that encourages personal independence in harmony with the environment.

Edited by Deborah Balmuth and Robin Catalano
Cover design by Carol Jessop, Black Trout Design
Cover and interior photographs by Giles Prett except those by
© Jeff Burke and Lorraine Triolo for Artville on pages 83 and 85;
© Eyewire Images on pages 17, 20, 82, 84, 97, 103, 120, and 134
Illustrations by Terry Dovaston
Text design and production by Mark Tomasi
Production assistance by Susan Bernier
Indexed by Barbara Hagerty

The information in this book is true and complete to the best of our knowledge. All recommendations are made without guarantee on the part of the author or Storey Books. The author and publisher disclaim any liability in connection with the use of this information. For additional information please contact Storey Books, Schoolhouse Road, Pownal, Vermont 05261.

Storey books are available for special premium and promotional uses and for customized editions. For further information, please call Storey's Custom Publishing Department at 1-800-793-9396.

Printed in the United States by Banta Book Group, Menasha, WI
10 9 8 7 6 5 4 3 2

Library of Congress Cataloging-in-Publication Data
Failor, Catherine.
    Making transparent soap : the art of crafting molding, scenting, and coloring / Catherine Failor.
        p.   cm.
    ISBN 1-58017-244-X (pbk. : alk. paper)
    1. Soap. I. Title.
TP991.F262   2000
668'.12—dc21

99-055700
CIP

Dedication

This book is for my parents, Letitia and the late Robert Failor, for their love and support.

Acknowledgments

Many, many thanks go to my good friend Kay Whaley, who has been a constant source of inspiration, ideas, and support throughout the writing of this book.

A grateful acknowledgment goes to Elaine White for her time and valuable suggestions.

A few years ago, when she started work on *The Natural Soap Book,* Susan Miller Cavitch called me up for help. What little help I could offer has been returned many times over through her kind encouragement. Thanks, Susan.

Thanks to John Toso at Sappo Hill, my best friend in the soap business.

To the Portland Public Library — I can't count the times I called the reference desk. What would life be without our libraries?

Many thank-yous to all these helpful people: Clyde Abston, Charlie Schmalz, Luis Spitz, George Whaley, Ed Paladini, Peter Cade, John Prutsman, Jim Bronner, Ken Peterson, and Peter Fox.

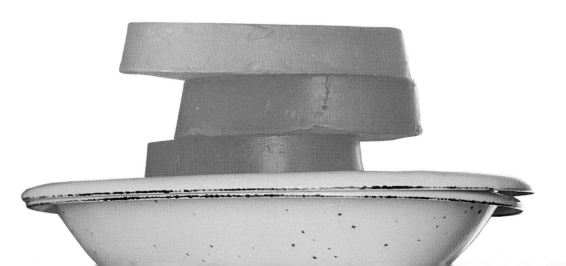

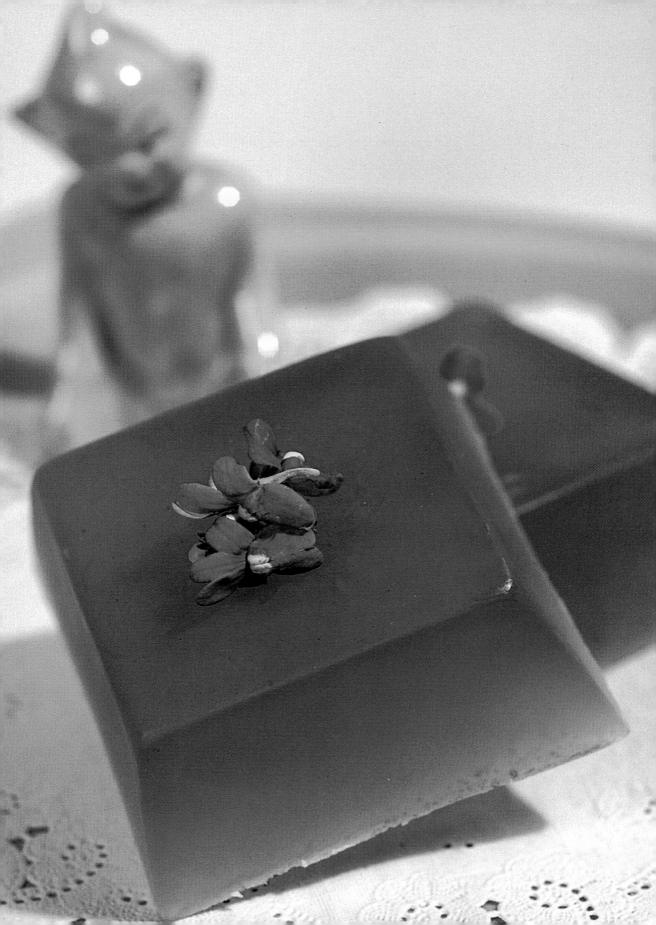

contents

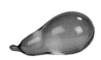
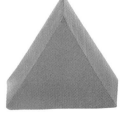

introduction

Zilch. That's how much informed, practical information on transparent soapmaking is currently available to the amateur soapmaker. Why? Not because the process requires a Ph.D. in chemistry or exotic and expensive chemical ingredients impossible for the layperson to obtain. It doesn't. If you can follow a recipe from a cookbook you can make transparent soap, and you don't need to look much further than your supermarket, drugstore, and liquor store for all the necessary ingredients.

Opaque soaps have been manufactured for at least two thousand years, but transparent soap is a relative newcomer — the first bars were produced almost exactly two hundred years ago. So information regarding its manufacture hasn't been circulating for as long or as widely as information concerning opaque soap. The descriptions that do exist are scanty and often confusing. And as is typical with many manufacturing processes, trade secrecy has constricted the informational flow down to a dribble. It's just not in the best interest of Neutrogena or Pear to publish a detailed treatise on transparent soapmaking.

I was in business 5 years as a soapmaker before attempting to make transparent soap. It was a bit overwhelming. All the information pertaining to the manufacture of transparent soap resembled a jigsaw puzzle with half of its pieces missing. But the challenge was there. Several months of trial-and-error experimentation ensued, and most batches ended up in the garbage can. Finally came the day when information and observation joined to create the big picture. That's what this book contains — all of the relevance with, I hope, none of the confusion.

Soapmaking is a lot like cooking. The ingredients are measured, mixed, heated, and poured into pans or molds. If your kitchen contains the basic utensils needed for cooking, you're all set. The spoons, whisks, spatulas, and pots used to make chicken soup or bake a chocolate cake can be used to make transparent soap. An accurate scale is something you might not have, but that can always be borrowed from a friend or purchased secondhand.

Transparent soap consists of the same base that opaque soap does — animal or vegetable oil combined with lye. Lye usually elicits a strong reaction from the uninitiated. "Lye??? You mean there's lye in soap? Lye is a poison!!!" But the chemical world is full of beasts turned beauties — it's just a matter of marrying well. Lye combined with oil is no longer lye, and oil combined with lye is no longer oil. Soap and glycerin are born.

Transparent soap contains a few things that opaque soap doesn't. These aren't mysterious chemicals with impossible-to-pronounce names. In fact, you're sure to have one of the ingredients sitting on your kitchen table — ordinary granulated sugar. Another additive, 190-proof grain alcohol, or ethanol, might be tucked away in the liquor cabinet. You probably won't have a bottle of glycerin on hand, but it's easily found at most drugstores.

I hope this will be enough to dispel any initial reluctance you might have about making transparent soap. After all, every bath and body retail chain on the planet is making it, so why don't you? I guarantee that handmade transparent soap will feel softer, richer, and creamier than any commercial brand on the market.

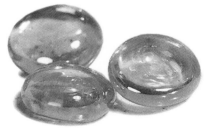

all about ① soap

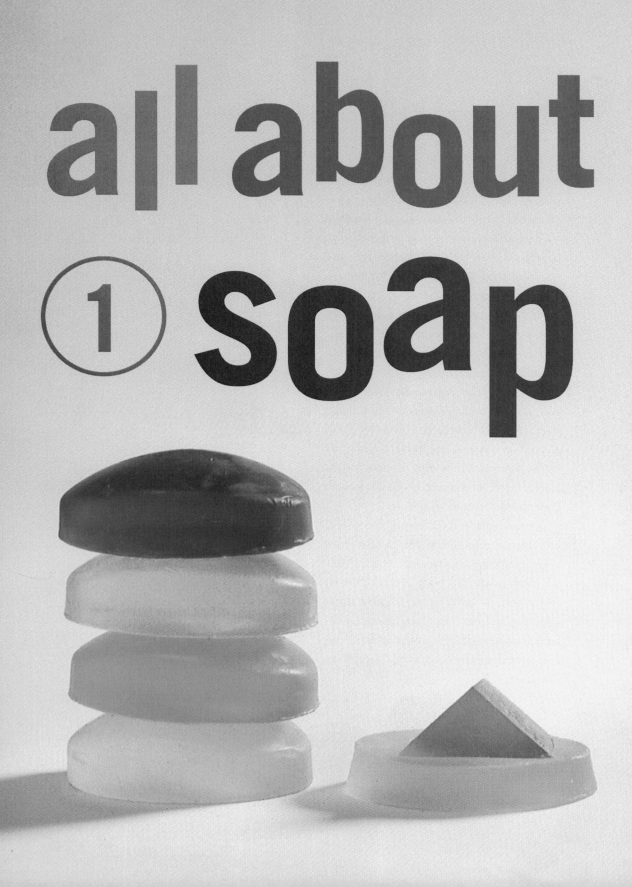

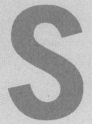**S**oapmaking is one of the oldest industries in the world, although no one really knows just when soap was discovered. The first reference to soap occurs in Sumerian clay tablets dated about 2500 B.C., but this was probably not a true soap. The early Romans used hot water and scraped their bodies with twigs or a special tool called a strigil. Some sources indicate that the Gauls were the first people to make soap and that the later Romans, during the conquests of Julius Caesar, learned the art from them. Excavations of ancient Pompeii reveal the presence of a soap factory.

Soapmaking as an art and science has been so refined that much modern "soap" is no longer soap in the true sense of the word. These soaps, which are actually synthetic detergents, became popular during World War II in response to a shortage of soapmaking oils. Many techniques now used by the home soapmaker are revivals of pre-twentieth century soapcrafting.

early soapmaking

Soap manufacture flourished in Europe from the eighth century onward in such towns as Castilla in Spain, Marseilles in France, and Savona in Italy.

The city name of Savona is the source of the names *savon, sabon,* and *jabon,* which mean "soap" in French, Portuguese, and Spanish, respectively. These earlier soaps were available only to the rich; it wasn't until the nineteenth century that soap of decent quality could be afforded by the common person.

Probably the first and certainly the best-known transparent soap is Pears. In 1798, Andrew Pears opened a barbershop in a fashionable London neighborhood. As business grew he began making his own creams, pomades, and powders. The soaps available at that time were often crude and quite alkaline, so Pears set about experimenting with his own formulas. He discovered that when he dissolved ordinary soap in alcohol, the resulting soap was both mild and transparent. Mass production began, and with the promotional help of his son-in-law, Thomas J. Barratt, sometimes called the father of advertising, Pears created a market that still retains a loyal following some two hundred years later.

▼ Soap can be produced in a variety of ways, but until now, home soapmakers used the cold-process method.

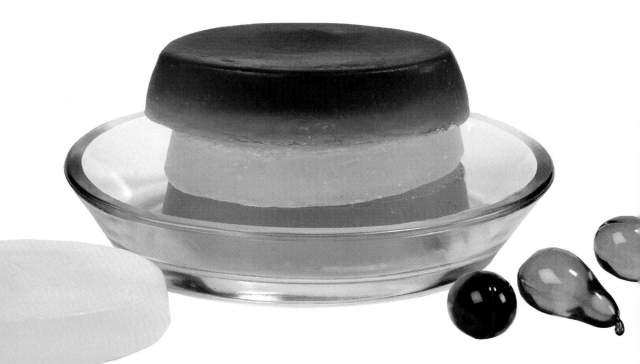

what is soap?

Soap is the by-product of a chemical reaction called saponification. Fatty acids present in either vegetable or animal oils are combined with a strong base, or alkali, namely caustic soda or caustic potash. Sodium-based (soda) soaps are hard; potassium-based (potash) soaps are liquid.

Large-scale commercial production of soap is done in enormous steam-heated vats by use of the full-boiled method. This process allows for the greatest control, because any unreacted lye can be removed at the end of the process. Some smaller specialty soap companies and the home soapmaker use the cold-process method, whereby the heat generated from the reaction of fatty acids and alkalis enables the soap to form. These soaps are usually less neutral than full-boiled soaps. Transparent soap is made by the semi-boiled method. The oils and caustic solution are combined and then heated, though not to the boiling point.

A neutral pH is 7. The pH of our skin ranges between 5 and 6.5, which is somewhat acidic. "Neutral" soaps are quite alkaline, with a pH of about 9.5. This wide discrepancy between our skin's pH and the pH of soap explains why so many soaps are drying to the skin.

This problem can be somewhat corrected by superfatting, or adding an excess of fatty acids or oils. Another process involves both superfatting the sodium soap and blending it with a soap created from the chemical compound called triethanolamine (TEA). The resulting soap is both extremely mild and easily rinsed off. The inventor of the process referred to this property as "neutrogenous," and that's how Neutrogena soap was born.

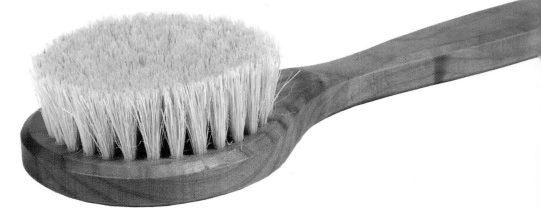

▲ A strong bristle brush helps exfoliate dead skin cells before washing.

How Does Soap Clean?

Soap has been cleansing us for centuries without anyone's knowing just how. The answer lies in the molecular structures of water, oil, and soap.

Water is a bipolar molecule. One of its ends, two hydrogen atoms, is positively charged; the other end, an oxygen atom, is negatively charged. This bipolar nature gives water a cohesiveness that resists being broken apart; you may have noticed that a drinking glass can be filled with water until the water is actually standing above the rim without overflowing. Water's love for itself makes it particularly incompatible with oil. This is because oil has an electrical charge that is uniform; there are no positive and negative poles to the molecule. What is needed to bring water and oil together is a substance that resembles them both — partly polar, partly nonpolar, able to act as an intermediary. That's what soap is.

During saponification, the fatty acids combine with the caustic sodium or potassium to form a soap molecule. One end of this molecule is composed of the water-soluble sodium or potassium group; the other end consists of the water-insoluble fatty acid group. This molecule looks like a snake, with a sodium "head" and a fatty acid "tail."

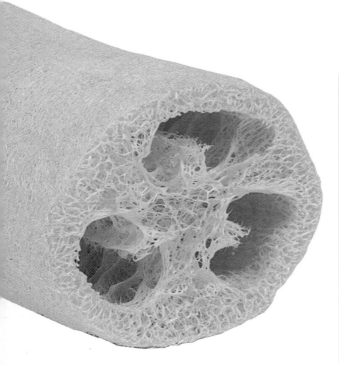

▲ A loofah sponge is made from the loofah gourd, a plant that grows in North America.

 UNIQUE QUALITIES OF TRANSPARENT SOAP

Because of the presence of additives, a transparent bar of soap contains only about 50 to 60 percent actual soap. Opaque bars contain approximately 85 percent. This difference explains why transparent bars have shorter life spans in your shower and sink. And even though both transparent soap and opaque soap have about the same pH, transparent soap rinses off the skin much more readily. This accounts for its exceptional mildness.

When soap is added to plain water, it doesn't actually dissolve. What happens is that the fatty tails hurry to the surface to avoid contact with the water and align themselves tail-up in the air. This breaks the water's surface tension and causes it to spread. If you take some soap solution and add it to that nearly overflowing glass of water, it will immediately cause the water to cascade over the rim of the glass.

Soil is usually enveloped in an oily film. When soiled fabrics or oils are added to soapy water, the fatty tails of the soap rush to them, seeking to bond with a substance of similar molecular makeup. These tails act as tiny hammers, chipping away at the soil and grease. The grease then balls up into smaller droplets. With the soap's oil-loving tails embedded in the grease and its water-loving sodium heads straining outward toward the water in the basin, the grease and grime can be washed down the drain.

Opaque Soap, Transparent Soap

During part of the soapmaking process, all soap passes through a colloidal phase. A colloid is any gel-like insoluble substance made up of particles larger than molecules but small enough so that they remain suspended in a fluid medium without settling to the bottom. If you've ever made soap and peeked at it while it is curing in the molds, you might have noticed that at one point the soap appears as a translucent gel. This is the colloidal state.

As the soap cools, long fibrous crystals begin developing. They increase in number and length and enmesh with one another. Gradually the translucency of the colloidal state disappears and the soap becomes opaque. This is because the

Throughout this book you'll find several safety precautions. In order to fully protect yourself during the soapmaking process, be sure to follow each caution carefully.

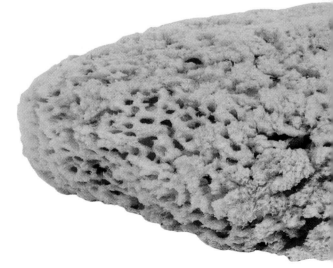

▲ A natural sea sponge offers a tight, yet absorbent, skin-scrubbing tool.

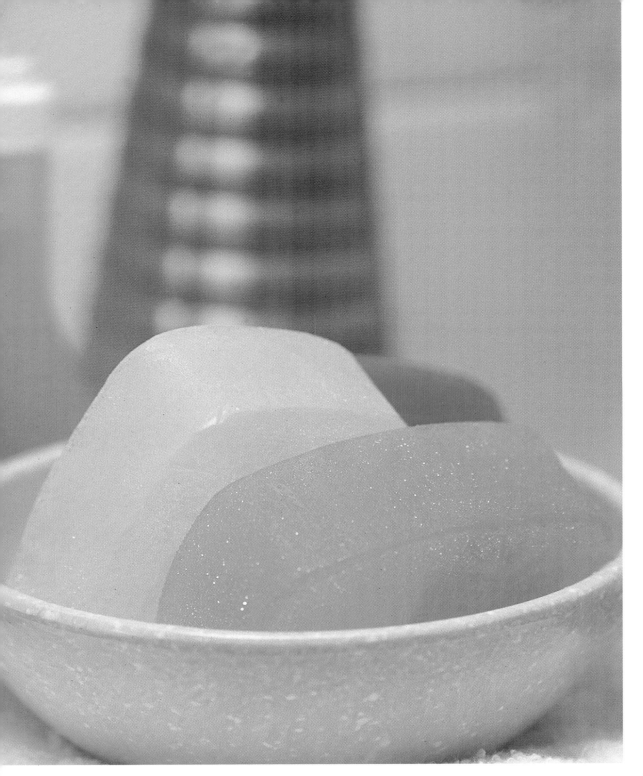

▲ Transparent soap, with its myriad colors, scents, and shapes, brightens any bathroom or kitchen.

increasing number of crystals renders the soap impervious to the passage of light waves. These crystals are what give ordinary bar soap its opacity.

Transparent soap is made by the same initial process as opaque soap. But at the point when the soap gels, solvents are added. Glycerin, ethyl alcohol (ethanol), and ordinary table sugar are the solvents described in this book. These solvents hold the soap mass in the colloidal state and suppress the development of long crystals. Transparent soap does contain crystals, but they are so exceedingly small that light waves can pass right through the bar. Transparency is defined as the ability to read 14-point typeface through a ¼" thick sliver of soap.

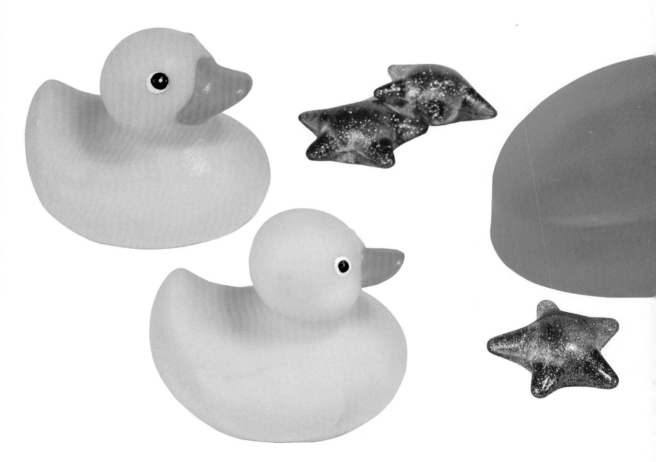

▲ **Make bathtime fun for both children and adults with the addition of tub toys, bath beads, and vibrant transparent soap.**

knowing ② your ingredients

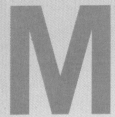**M**ost of the things we're surrounded with in our lives are so commonplace that we rarely stop to consider just what they really are made of. This is especially true in the modern industrialized world, because almost all of our material goods are made by a machine or another person, usually thousands of miles away. But whether you're baking bread, glazing pottery, or building a cabinet, success always hinges on a knowledge of each material's characteristics and how one material affects another.

Soapmaking is no different. Each fat and oil used to produce a bar of soap has its own unique chemistry, which affects the soap's hardness, solubility, and lather. This chapter is intended to deepen your understanding of each ingredient's characteristics, which will be useful for problem solving or for formulating your own soap. Chapters 4–6 contain charts and further information on soapmaking.

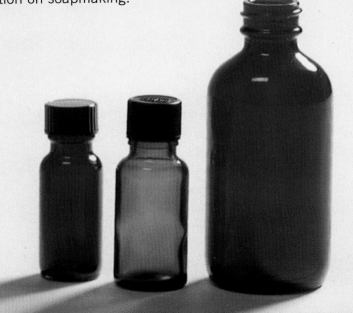

fats and oils

The difference between a fat and an oil is somewhat arbitrary and is based on physical state at room temperature — fat is solid; oil is liquid.

Oils are divided into three classes: mineral oils (derived from petroleum), essential oils (any volatile oil that gives a distinctive fragrance to a plant, flower, or fruit), and fixed oils. Fixed oils, which are either animal or vegetable in origin, constitute the main raw materials for soapmaking because of their easy reactivity with alkalis. Specifically, the fatty acids in these oils are what combine chemically with the alkalis; this process is known as saponification. The fixed oils are further classified as follows:

Hard fats are largely composed of stearin and palmitin, fatty acids that are solid at room temperature and therefore lend firmness to the fats; this firmness, however, means that soaps created from hard fats do not readily dissolve in water. A soap composed exclusively of either palm oil or tallow will be very brittle, with a low but persistent lather.

Palm oil and animal tallow are the two most common hard fats used for soapmaking. Palm oil is extracted from the fruit pulp of the oil palm and is becoming increasingly difficult to find in the United States because of health concerns over saturated fats in our diets. Wholesale bakery or grocery suppliers are the most likely sources for 35-pound pails. Other suppliers are listed in Resources.

Tallow is the fat of cattle or sheep; suet is the fat specifically surrounding the kidneys of these animals. Tallow and palm oil can be used interchangeably in soap formulation, although tallow may worsen skin conditions such as eczema and acne. It has been the primary fat used in soapmaking for two millennia and is much easier to obtain than palm oil. Simple instructions for rendering tallow are outlined on the facing page.

▼ An oil is a type of fat that is liquid at room temperature.

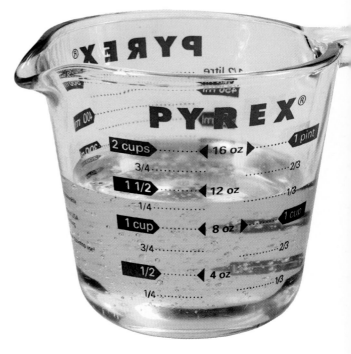

Rendering Tallow

If you haven't any philosophical objections to animal-based soap, you can use lard, which is found in 1-pound blocks at your grocery, or you can render tallow. Rendering needs to be done a day before soapmaking.

Tallow can be purchased from butchers or from rendering plants. It usually comes in large slabs, though some butchers grind it up into hamburger consistency for customers with bird feeders. Hamburger consistency is ideal; the smaller the pieces, the faster the rendering time. Buy more fat than the recipe calls for, since there are some impurities that will be discarded after rendering. If a recipe calls for 2 pounds of tallow, buy 3. And as long as you're going through the trouble of rendering, make some extra now if you'll be mixing more soap in the future. It keeps indefinitely in the freezer.

To render, chop the tallow into small chunks. In a large pot, bring to a boil a few cups of water. (Some opaque soapmaking books call for salted water, but salt can cause cloudiness in transparent soap.) Add the fat carefully to avoid splashing. Stirring occasionally, bring the water back up to a boil, then turn the heat to low, and cover the pot. Depending on the amount of fat being rendered, it may take a few hours until all the fat has melted. If you're impatient, you can expedite the process by chopping up the hot chunks of fat in a blender or food processor.

WHAT ABOUT LARD?

As an alternative to palm oil and tallow, lard can be used. Lard is rendered pig fat. One big advantage of lard is that you can buy it cheaply in 1-pound cubes at most grocery stores, already cleaned and refined. Soap made with lard is a bit softer than soap made with palm oil or tallow.

Once the fat has completely melted, pour it through a large strainer and into another pot or bowl; toss out any of the impurities that might be left in the strainer. Let the fat cool to room temperature, then set it in the refrigerator overnight. By the next day, the fat will have cooled into three layers: white tallow on top, a middle grayish granular layer, and water or gel on the bottom. Lift the disc of tallow, and scrape away all of the gray layer adhering to it.

This disc of white tallow will soon be transformed into a clear, jewel-like bar of transparent soap.

Nut Oils

Coconut oil and palm kernel oil are the most typical nut oils used for soapmaking. Coconut and palm kernel oils are characterized by a large proportion of lauric acid, which produces a very soluble and quick-lathering soap. (Not all nut oils have this high percentage of lauric acid.) What is unusual about lauric acid is that it also produces a hard soap; all other oils capable of hardening soap have the disadvantage of poor solubility. Soaps created exclusively from coconut or palm kernel oil, however, are drying to the skin, and though they lather profusely, the lather is short-lived.

▼ **One of the most popular oils for soapmaking is created from the common coconut.**

Coconut oil is pressed from dried coconut meat (copra), and palm kernel oil is extracted from the kernel (as opposed to the fruit) of the oil palm. Coconut oil can be purchased at most health food stores; 35-pound pails can also be found at large grocery wholesalers or bakery supply houses. Palm kernel oil is not as easy to find. For more information, consult Resources.

Both of these oils have similar soapmaking properties and can be used interchangeably. However, more sodium hydroxide is necessary to saponify coconut oil than is needed for palm kernel oil. The recipes in this book have been calculated for coconut oil only. If you wish to use palm kernel oil in place of coconut oil, see Formulating Opaque and Transparent Soap in chapter 5 and recalculate. Palm kernel oil requires approximately 80 percent of the amount of sodium hydroxide needed to saponify coconut oil.

Soft Oils

Unsaturated fatty acids, such as oleic acid and linoleic acid, are the primary components of most soft oils: olive, cottonseed, corn, canola, soybean, sesame, and peanut oils are common soft oils. The soapmaking properties of these oils vary according to the proportions of each oil's fatty acid content, but generally soft oils yield thin, long-lasting lathers with good detergent properties. None of these oils should be used alone for soapmaking, however, as they cannot produce a hard bar.

> **Note:** Avoid sulfonated castor oil, which is water soluble; this will cause an oil blend to "seize" and curdle as soon as the lye solution is added.

▼ Although soft oils are not used alone in transparent soapmaking, they lend valuable lathering and detergent properties to the finished product.

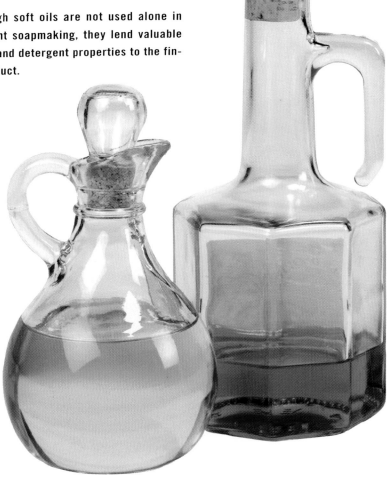

Castor oil, a thick, viscous oil extracted from the castor bean, is the traditional soft oil of choice for transparent soapmaking. Castor oil differs from most other soft oils in its fatty acid composition; 80 to 85 percent of castor oil is ricinoleic acid. The peculiar nature of this fatty acid gives castor solventlike properties, and solvents are what render ordinary soap transparent. Other soft oils can be substituted for castor oil, but the resulting soap will be somewhat less transparent.

Castor oil has the additional virtue of acting as a humectant: it draws and holds moisture from the air to the skin. Too large a proportion of castor oil in a recipe, however, makes the finished bar soft and sticky and reduces its lathering properties. Castor oil can be found in or ordered from drugstores and health food stores. Other sources are listed in the back of this book.

Blending Oils

You can see from the previous description of oils that any single oil used alone will not produce a satisfactory bar of soap — the soap will be too hard, too soft, or of insufficient lather. One of the arts of soapmaking lies in the selection and blending of oils. The best soap consists of coconut or palm kernel oil for firmness and quick foam; a hard fat for firmness and for stabilizing and extending the life of the lather; and a soft oil for a rich, soluble lather. For readers who are interested in formulating their own soaps, chapter 5 contains additional information. Consult the chart on the facing page for at-a-glance information on the different fats and oils.

▼ **Castor oil creates a rich, creamy lather and helps moisturize the skin.**

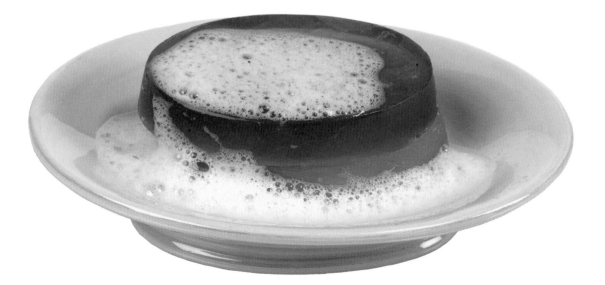

Properties of Common Oils and Fats

Soap Made from	Color	Consistency	Lather	Cleansing Properties	Action on Skin	How Saponified
Castor Oil	Pale yellow	Soft	Thick, lasting	Fair	Mild	Easily
Coconut Oil	Pale yellow to white	Extremely hard	Quick, foamy, large bubbles; does not last	Excellent	Biting action; roughens skin	Quickly
Cotton-seed Oil	Buff to bright yellow	Medium to soft	Oily, abundant, medium lasting	Good	Mild	Fairly easily
Lard	White	Hard	Fairly slow, lasting, thick	Good	Very mild	Fairly easily
Olive Oil	Shades of green	Very soft	Oily, close, lather persists	Very fair	Very mild	Fairly easily
Palm Kernel Oil	Pale yellow to white	Extremely hard	Quick, foamy, large bubbles; does not last	Excellent	Biting action; roughens skin	Quickly
Palm Oil	Buff	Very hard	Slow, lasting, close	Very good	Very mild	Very easily
Rosin	Yellow to dark brown	Soft	Oily, thick	Fair	Mild	Quickly
Soybean Oil	Pale yellow to dull white	Soft	Oily, abundant, medium lasting	Fair	Mild	Fairly easily
Tallow	Pale buff to white	Very hard	Fairly slow, lasting, thick	Good	Very mild	Fairly easily

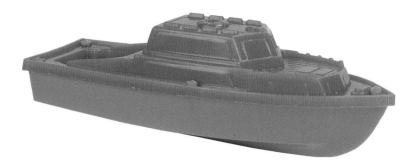

other ingredients

Since soap consists of an oil-and-water bond, certain ingredients are needed to help form this bond.

Alkalis

The two alkalis used in soap production are sodium hydroxide, also called lye or caustic soda, and potassium hydroxide, or caustic potash. Soda-based soaps are solid; potash-based soaps are liquid. Caustic soda is used for all the transparent soap recipes in this book.

Commercially, caustic soda is produced by the electrolysis of brine (seawater); the other by-product of this process is chlorine, used for bleaching and water treatment. Caustic soda is most frequently found in either bead or flake form; large soap operations purchase it as a liquid. You can find pure lye in 12-ounce cans in the cleaning section of your local supermarket; look for Red Devil brand. Don't use Drano; it's not pure lye. If you plan to make a lot of soap, the cheapest and easiest alternative is a 50-pound bag, which can be purchased from chemical wholesalers in your area. Other sources of caustic soda are listed in Resources.

Caustic soda is extremely hygroscopic, or water-loving; a small bead will quickly swell up with atmospheric moisture and become a large droplet. Care must therefore be taken in storing any half-used containers. Caustic soda is also extremely corrosive — it burns skin within seconds of exposure. Gloves and goggles are a must during the handling and mixing of lye solutions and during the mixing of the soap itself.

IN CASE OF ACCIDENTAL EXPOSURE TO LYE

In case of exposure of lye to the skin, always keep a bottle of vinegar or lemon juice handy — the strong acid quickly neutralizes the strong base of lye. This works faster than rinsing with plain water, but don't use vinegar or lemon juice in the eyes or if the lye has been ingested — seek immediate medical attention. The rule for caustic soda is the same as that for any hazardous substance: read the warning labels!

Distilled or Soft Water

Whether you're making transparent or opaque soap, water will be mixed with caustic soda to create a lye solution.

Transparent soaps require additional water in the form of a sugar solution. Tap water is not recommended; depending upon where you live, it can contain dissolved salts and other mineral impurities that may impart a cloudiness or "efflorescence," as transparent soapmakers say, to the finished bar of soap. These salts and minerals act as "seeds" around which other impurities can coalesce, much as pearls form around grains of sand inside an oyster. For this reason, distilled or soft water is strongly recommended for transparent soap.

Water also contributes to the soap's transparency because of its nature as a solvent. Even though much of this water eventually evaporates, the soap retains its transparency.

▶ **Water is an essential ingredient in any soap recipe. Use distilled or soft water for best results.**

Alcohol

Alcohol is the primary solvent used in transparent soapmaking. After the initial batch of soap has been mixed and left to sit in the pot for a couple of hours, alcohol is added. With a little stirring, the alcohol dissolves the soap into a clear, amber liquid. Some old soap manuals claim that it's possible to make transparent soap without alcohol; additional glycerin and sugar solution are used instead. But a soap made without alcohol will likely cloud with age.

Ethyl alcohol (or ethanol), more commonly known as 190-proof grain alcohol, is the type of alcohol required for all the recipes in this book. Ethanol, colorless and extremely flammable, is produced by the fermentation of starches, sugars, and other carbohydrates. Less expensive isopropyl alcohol can be substituted for a certain amount of ethanol. (Isopropyl alcohol is prepared from propylene, a gas obtained during the refinement of petroleum.) But because ethanol is a stronger solvent than isopropyl alcohol, soap made with an ethanol/isopropyl blend will be less transparent.

Ethanol can be purchased through scientific and chemical supply houses. It is referred to as denatured, and it costs considerably less than liquor store ethanol, particularly when you purchase by the

▼ **Being creative when choosing scents, colors, and molds for your soaps will turn the predictable into the unexpected.**

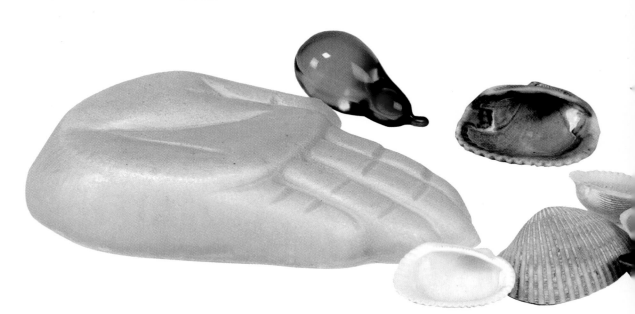

gallon. The trick is to find it in your local area. Although some suppliers are listed in Resources, shippers such as United Parcel Service consider ethanol a hazardous substance owing to its flammability. An extra fee (besides the shipping cost) is consequently added to the denatured alcohol. Its cost may then end up equaling or even exceeding the cost of liquor store ethanol. To find denatured alcohol in your hometown, look in the yellow pages under Scientific Instruments and Supplies or Chemicals.

Ethanol is denatured to make it unfit for drinking or redistillation. Many substances are used as denaturants — essential oils, ketones, vinegar, benzene, bone oil — to name just a few. Many of these denaturants are either toxic or strong-smelling, making them unsuitable for soapmaking.

Two denatured alcohols that are acceptable for use in soaps and shampoos are SDA 3A and SDA 3C. SDA stands for Specially Denatured Alcohol. SDA 3A is composed of 100 parts ethanol to 5 parts methyl alcohol. SDA 3C is 100 parts ethanol to 5 parts isopropyl alcohol. So when ordering denatured ethanol, be sure to specify either SDA 3A or 3C.

WHERE TO BUY ETHANOL

Ethanol can be found at your local supermarket or liquor store. The most common brand names are Clear Springs and Everclear. When purchasing bottles for soapmaking, keep in mind that 1 fluid pint of alcohol doesn't weigh 1 pound; alcohol has a lower specific gravity than water. One pint of alcohol weighs roughly 12.5 ounces.

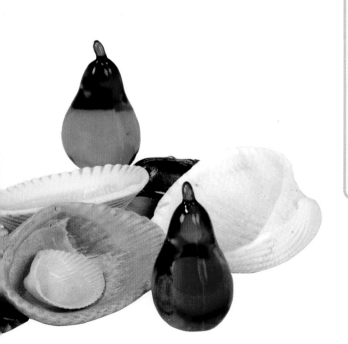

Glycerin

The term *glycerin soap* has come to be synonymous with transparent soap even though transparent soap can be made without it. Nonetheless, most of the recipes in this book do include glycerin. Not only is glycerin an excellent solvent, but, like castor oil, it acts as an emollient and a humectant, drawing moisture from the air and holding it to the skin. When glycerin is used in excess, however, its humectant properties can cause a bar of soap to "sweat."

Glycerin is actually an alcohol. Sweet and very viscous, it is a naturally occurring by-product of saponification. The reaction of a fatty acid and an alkali creates soap and glycerin, the percentage of glycerin being between 10 and 13 percent. In homemade soap production, glycerin is retained in the bar. Large soap manufacturers extract it and sell it as a

When ordering glycerin and castor oil from scientific supply houses, ask for the technical grade, which is less expensive than the reagent grade.

valuable raw material. Synthetic glycerin, or propylene glycol, is derived from propylene, a by-product of petroleum distillation.

Glycerin can be found or ordered from drugstores and health food stores. Scientific supply houses are another source. Look in Resources for more information.

▼ **The use of glycerin will help produce soap bars that are crystal clear.**

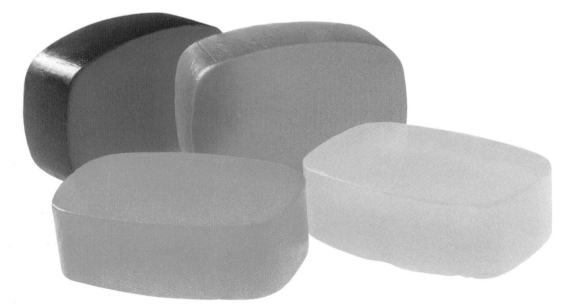

Sugar

The virtues of ordinary table sugar, or sucrose, in the making of transparent soap can't be overemphasized. Many formulations using only alcohol and glycerin for transparency often produce a slightly cloudy bar; a touch of sugar solution renders these same formulations perfectly transparent. Another virtue of sugar is its inexpensiveness. It can be used as a partial substitute for the more costly alcohol and glycerin.

Too much sugar in the soap, however, causes stickiness and sweatiness — the same problem encountered with an excess of glycerin. And although sugar produces even greater transparency than glycerin, it lacks the humectant and emollient properties of glycerin.

Never substitute powdered sugar for granulated sugar — it contains cornstarch, which will ruin your soap's transparency.

Rosin

Rosin, or resin, is the residue left after the volatile oils have been distilled from the oleoresin of pine trees. Rosin comes in the form of transparent, pale yellow lumps. In soap formulations, it changes color and, depending upon the percentage used, it can create a deep root beer–colored bar.

Rosin is not a crucial ingredient in transparent soapmaking, though it was quite popular with old-time soapmakers. Besides its excellent transparency-producing properties, it imparts a rich creamy finish to the soap, has a wonderful fragrance, and prevents rancidity. Too much rosin can soften and cloud the soap.

▼ **A small amount of granulated table sugar can work wonders in clarifying soap mixtures that are too cloudy.**

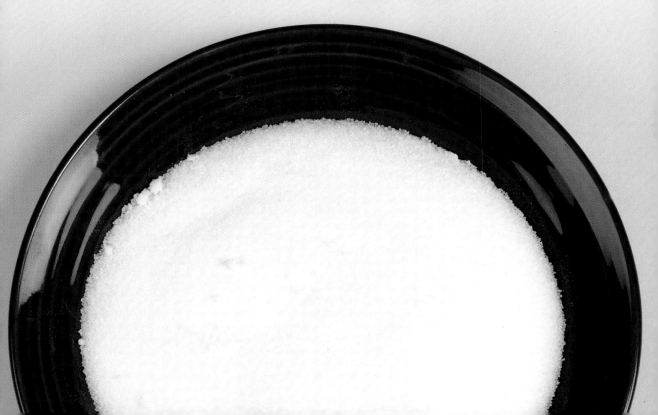

Stearic Acid

Stearic acid, or stearin, is a fatty acid derived from palm oil, tallow, and other sources. Although some of the recipes in this book call for it, stearic acid isn't an essential ingredient for transparent soapmaking. However, it does have some special uses. Because it is a free fatty acid, it provides an easy way to adjust the soap's pH if the soap is too alkaline. It can be used as a substitute for palm oil and tallow. A small quantity of stearic acid added to an oil blend hastens saponification, cutting down on stirring time. It also makes a harder bar of soap.

Other fatty acids, such as oleic acid, can be used, but stearic acid has a couple of advantages. It is relatively odorless, which isn't true of oleic acid and some of the other fatty acids, and it is easier to find.

Stearic acid comes as a white, waxy flake. Scientific supply houses carry it. It may also be found in craft outlets that sell candle-making supplies, since stearic acid is often blended with paraffin wax to produce a slower-burning candle. Other sources are listed in Resources.

▼ **Using stearic acid in small quantities will help speed up the stirring process and make firmer bars of soap.**

Preservatives

Oils eventually turn rancid from oxidation. The unsaturated soft oils are more easily oxidized than are saturated oils, such as coconut and palm oils. Transparent soaps seem much less prone to rancidity than opaque soaps, perhaps because of the presence of alcohol, glycerin, and sugar, which all have preservative properties.

Rosin acts as a preservative, so the two rosin recipes in this book need no additional preservatives. If you are at all concerned about rancidity in the other recipes, mixed-tocopherol vitamin E is both natural and easily obtainable. Vitamin E is made up of several constituents, called tocopherols. Alpha-tocopherols specifically aid in healing skin, but there are many other types of tocopherols, such as beta and gamma. Mixed tocopherols are particularly effective antioxidants.

Like vitamin E, rosemary extract possesses superior preservative properties. For a 12-pound batch of soap, 2 or 3 tablespoons of either of these oils should be sufficient. Add them along with color and fragrance right before pouring the soap into molds.

> **Suppliers of natural preservatives, such as mixed-tocopherol vitamin E and rosemary extract, are listed in Resources.**

▼ **Easy-to-find vitamin E will help stave off soap rancidity by acting as a preservative.**

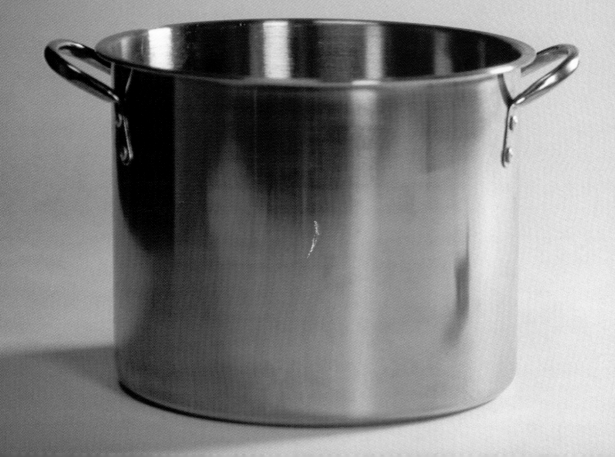

equipment
③ & safety
precautions

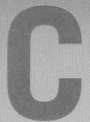Contrary to popular belief, making homemade soap doesn't require loads of special equipment and supplies or overly complex preparation methods. All you need are some essential pieces of equipment, inexpensive supplies, and basic know-how, and you're on your way to creating your own personalized soaps.

Many inexperienced — as well as some experienced — soapmakers find transparent soapmaking daunting. The double boilers. The higher temperatures and longer cook times. The alcohol and safety precautions. The extra steps (compared to cold processing). All I can say is: patience! With just a little practice, making transparent soap becomes familiar, easy, and fun.

basic equipment

The equipment necessary for making transparent soap is fairly basic. Almost everything is probably in your kitchen; if not, it can be borrowed from a friend or neighbor.

If you pour soap regularly and want to eliminate some of the hand labor, or if you desire more finished-looking wire-cut bars, chapter 7 contains instructions for building two inexpensive devices that are guaranteed to simplify your soapmaking.

Scales

Soapmaking is more akin to baking than to cooking. Cooking can be improvisational, and a good cook often relies more on inspiration than on written instruction. But correct measurements in baking and soapmaking spell the difference between success and failure.

▶ **A reliable kitchen scale is an indispensible tool. Look for a scale that can measure up to 20 pounds.**

Unless you can borrow one, an accurate scale will be your most expensive investment. All ingredients except color and fragrance need precise measurement. The scale must be able to register increments as small as 1 ounce, and should preferably be able to weigh up to 20 pounds. It might be worth your while to look around in secondhand shops and flea markets for used scales, but make sure you can test them with an object of known weight. Or look under Scales in the yellow pages. Many businesses carry used, reconditioned scales.

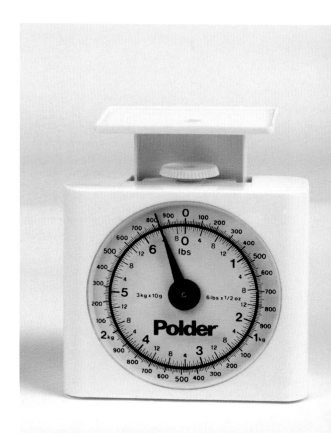

Mixing Pot

A 2- or 3-gallon pot (8 to 12 quarts) is an appropriate size for mixing the recipes in this book. If you want to double any recipes, a 4-gallon pot will be necessary. Whichever size you choose, the pot must be either stainless steel or enamel, since lye corrodes most other pots. If you put lye in an aluminum pot, the pot fizzes and turns dull gray. Enamel pots should be free of any rust. Rust in solution may cause cloudiness and mar the soap's overall transparency in the same way that mineralized water can.

Thermometer

Your thermometer must be able to measure up to 160°F (70°C). A glass candy thermometer or a deep-fry thermometer with a stainless steel stem is best.

Goggles and Gloves

These items are a must for mixing the lye solution and stirring the soap. Use rubber bands to secure the tops of the gloves around your arms.

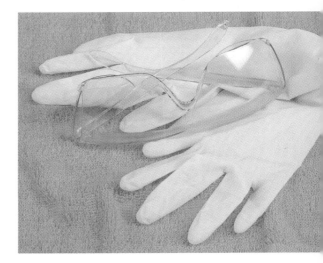

▶ **Top: A 3-gallon stainless-steel pot. Middle: A candy thermometer. Bottom: Surgical gloves and plastic goggles.**

Containers

You'll need a few miscellaneous containers for your sugar solution, glycerin, and alcohol. Plastic and glass are both fine choices. Quart-sized mayonnaise or cottage cheese containers work well.

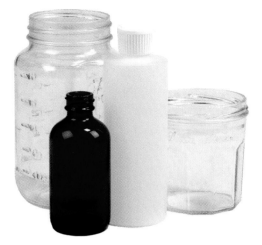

Stirrers and Mixers

For manual mixing, spatulas, stainless steel spoons, and wooden spoons work well. Whisks do the best job, particularly when you are stirring the alcohol into the soap. This dissolves the soap more completely; undissolved soap can mar the transparency.

Or try some of those miracles of the machine age. Blenders and food processors are fabulous devices for thickening the oil-lye mix in a matter of minutes, though they don't work for every phase of transparent soapmaking. You can also use a stick blender or electric hand-held mixer, preferably secondhand, so as to avoid soaping up your favorite kitchen model. Not only do hand-held electric mixers and stick blenders eliminate manual labor, but the increased agitation thickens the soap solution more quickly. Take care to start on low speed to avoid splashing.

Instructions and diagrams for constructing a very handy mixer out of an electric drill are given on pages 101–103. This mixer is useful for every phase of transparent soapmaking and will simplify the task considerably.

▼ **A stainless-steel whisk and spoon and a wooden spoon are essential stirring tools.**

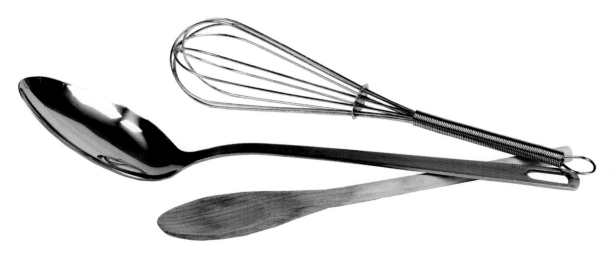

Plastic Sheeting

Plastic sheeting will be needed for covering the soap pot after adding the alcohol. Saran Wrap and other kitchen films aren't heavy enough. Use heavy-duty plastic film, approximately 3 to 4 ml thick, which can be found in the painting supply section of your local hardware store. Clear plastic is best. The soap solution can then be watched as it mixes in the pot.

Plastic sheeting is also a necessary item for lining a wooden mold. *Warning:* Don't line wooden molds with used plastic. Transparent soap has the viscosity of water when it is first poured and, like water, it seeps out of the tiniest hole.

Bungee Cords or Flexible Rope

You'll use bungee cords or flexible rope to secure the plastic sheeting to the top of the mixing pot. Both are inexpensive and can be found at any hardware store.

▼ ▶ **Plastic sheeting, bungee cords, and a sharp kitchen knife are supplies you may already have on hand.**

Cutters and Rulers

Any sharp kitchen knife will work for carving blocks of soap into bars. Or try using a square pastry blade or a stiff, 4" paint scraper; these two tools are pressed down into the soap to achieve a cleaner-looking cut. To create bars of uniform size, measure and score a grid on the top of the slab, then cut.

A hardened slab of transparent soap has a slightly uneven, pockmarked surface when first unmolded. This forms when small air bubbles present in the hot solution float up and imprint themselves on the cooling surface. A long-bladed knife or metal ruler works well for skimming off these irregularities. Another good scraping (and cutting) tool is a strip of sheet metal. You can get strips free by calling around to sheet metal shops — they usually have bins of odd-sized scraps that are otherwise bound for recycling. A piece 2" wide by 16" to 18" long is ideal, being both flexible and very easy to handle.

Molds

Transparent soap lends itself to a wide variety of molding possibilities. Molds made of flexible materials, such as plastic and rubber, work best. If the soap sticks to a less flexible mold, immerse the mold in hot water for a few seconds. This will slightly melt the soap away from the mold's surface. Always make sure that the top of the mold is as wide as or wider than the bottom, and be aware of any relief on the sides that could prevent the soap from releasing.

Look around your house for mold ideas. There are many options: tennis ball cans, plastic tofu trays, decorative plastic cookie box inserts, tart tins, milk cartons. Plastic sheeting draped into a shoebox or a cardboard box works fine. Or purchase a few plastic kitchen trays used for storing leftovers.

Some are even divided up into bar-sized compartments. If you want fancy molds, pay a visit to your local craft or ceramic supply store — you should be able to find the ubiquitous seashells, scallops, and other familiar designs. Kitchen accessory shops are another source. Metal molds, even aluminum ones, will not be a problem, since transparent soap is neutral when poured. Whatever you end up using, just check for any holes!

A simple wooden mold can be constructed in no time — you probably have enough scrap lumber in your garage or workshop to do the job.

▼ **Flexible material is necessary for soap molds; plastic is an excellent choice.**

WOODEN SOAP MOLD

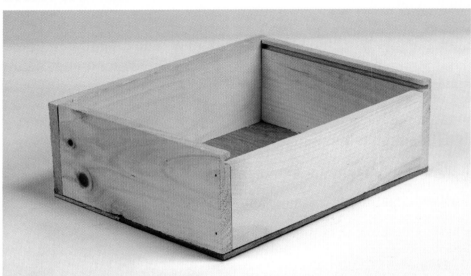

Materials:
- ⇨ 1 piece of plywood or particle board, ½–¾" thick and 14" x 14" square
- ⇨ Two 1" x 3" or 1" x 4" fir or pine boards
- ⇨ 36 1½" screws or nails
- ⇨ 1 piece plastic sheeting, 1–2 ml and 24" square
- ⇨ vegetable oil or glycerin

To make an easy mold for a 12-pound batch of soap:

1. If necessary, cut the piece of plywood or particleboard into a square measuring 14" x 14".

2. For the sides, cut the pine boards into two pieces 12" long and two pieces 13½" long.

3. Screw or nail the side boards into the plywood and into each other where they abut.

4. To eliminate most of the big creases in the plastic that will otherwise impress themselves into the hardened slab, brush the bottom and sides of the mold with vegetable oil or a bit of glycerin. This will create a tacky surface to which the plastic will adhere.

5. Line the mold with plastic sheeting before pouring the soap, making sure the plastic drapes a few inches over the sides. Lay the plastic in the mold, and smooth and flatten the creases.

The approximate yield for each recipe in this book is 11 to 12 pounds of soap. This will fill the wooden mold to a depth of approximately 2".

alcohol: safety procedures

It's very important to become familiar with the potential hazards of alcohol. This applies *especially* to anyone using gas heat. Alcohol must be kept away from open flames. For this reason, using a gas stove to process your soap is not recommended. Alcohol should pose no problem with electric ranges, however, unless spilled directly onto a heating element.

Ethanol is very flammable. It's particularly problematic because when it is ignited, the flame is sometimes difficult to see. A few precautions and some common sense should safeguard your work area or kitchen against accidents.

▶ **Before beginning to make soap, it is essential to equip your craft area with a working fire extinguisher. Accidents are rare, but you should be prepared.**

▶ **Equip the kitchen or work area with a fire extinguisher,** preferably an all-purpose 2A-10B:C. If you don't want to purchase or borrow an extinguisher, water will work. Alcohol is soluble in water, so water actually dilutes the burning alcohol. Apply the water as a spray, either out of a spray bottle or from the hose on your sink. Aim the spray at the base of the flames.

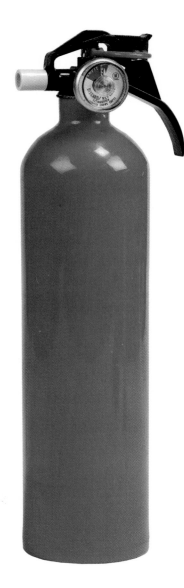

▶ Make sure the work area has adequate ventilation:

fans or open windows, and/or an exhaust vent over the range. You want to avoid a buildup of vapors; they may pose a fire hazard and cause dizziness if inhaled.

▶ Avoid the use of under-sized pots for mixing soap.

Allow at least 2" of headroom after the addition of alcohol and glycerin to ensure against any spillage. Keep electric mixers on medium-low speed. Even after the glycerin and sugar solution are added, a soap broth containing alcohol is still quite flammable.

▶ Adhere to all safety precautions.

These precautions are not intended to cause undue panic. Just as with the use of caustic soda, anyone exercising reasonable care with alcohol will have no problems. No soapmaking procedures involve pure, unmixed alcohol coming near a flame; any problems will be encountered after the alcohol has been stirred into solution with the soap. And since the alcohol is diluted in this form, it is substantially less flammable. Your soap pot will also be covered.

Only once in 3 years of transparent soapmaking have I had any trouble. While attending to another project, I absentmindedly left soap heating on the gas range. It boiled over, and the soap running down the sides ignited. There wasn't much actual spillage, so the fire was easily contained. I was lucky.

If you do have a gas range and are nervous about fire hazards, use an electric hot plate instead. Just make sure that it's in good condition, and plug it directly into the wall outlet and not into a small extension cord. Otherwise, you'll just be creating further fire hazards.

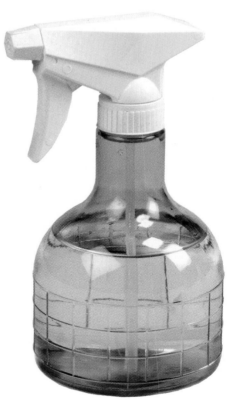

▶ **Water is important to have on hand, since it can dilute any burning alcohol. Use a spray bottle or your sink sprayer to dispense the water.**

making transparent

⑷ **soap**

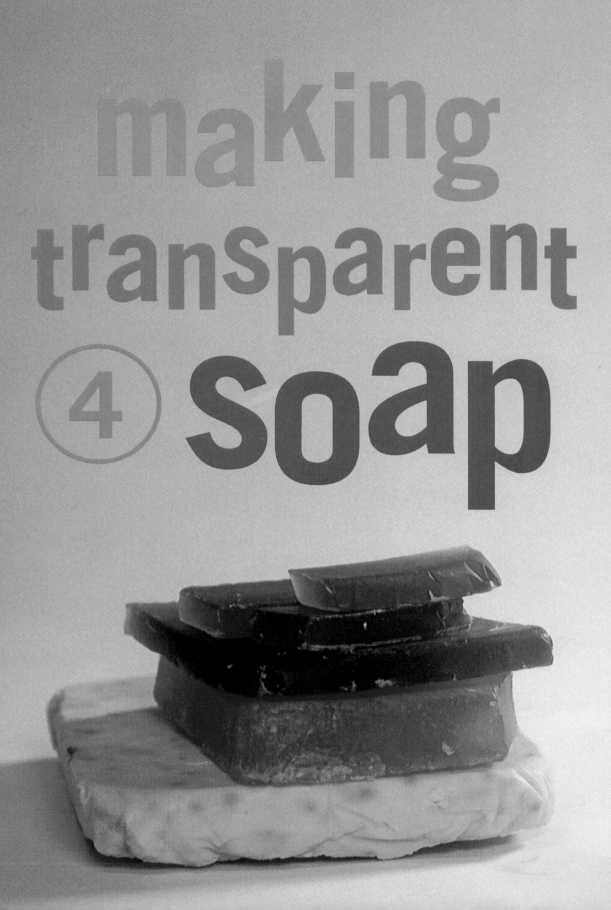

Early transparent soaps were manufactured by dissolving flaked toilet soap in vats of boiling alcohol. The broth was kept boiling until the bulk of the alcohol evaporated out of solution; this alcohol was condensed and reused in other batches. Dye and fragrance were stirred into the remaining broth, which was then poured into molds for cooling.

After the hardened blocks of soap were removed from the molds and cut, the bars were placed into a warm, well-ventilated room for weeks, even months. One old recipe called for a drying time of 1 year!

Luckily, transparent soapmaking is much easier today. The procedures and photos in this chapter offer a clear, simple method for making your own transparent soap. The first technique outlined is the paste method, the basic soapmaking technique. For an easy alternative to part of this procedure (one which avoids tracing and stirring), see The Alcohol/Lye Method on page 56.

basic paste method

1 Measure All Ingredients

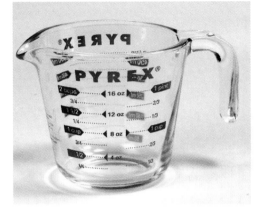

2 Prepare the Lye Solution

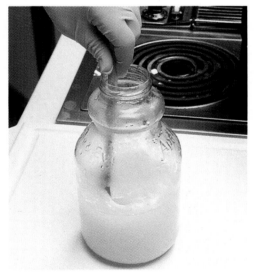

Precise measurements are a must for the lye solution. It's amazing what a difference it makes to your finished bar if the solution is a bit weak or a bit strong.

A half-gallon or 1-gallon glass jar works well for mixing the water and soda beads. If the jar has a lid, pierce two small holes on opposite sides of the lid, using an ice pick or screwdriver. The lye solution can then be added to the oil in a thin stream, ensuring more thorough mixing.

Enamel, stainless steel, glazed ceramic, and plastic are also suitable for containing a hot lye solution. The plastic must be the heavier kind — the same thickness as a 5-gallon paint container or laundry detergent pail. Never use aluminum, as explained earlier. Also, make sure these containers have at least 3 to 4 inches headroom for stirring.

➲ With gloves and goggles on, measure the water and the soda beads separately. Use room-temperature distilled water.

➲ Mix together, stir vigorously, and avoid inhaling the fumes. The temperature of the water will rise to 200°F (92°C) moments after the addition of the caustic soda. *Be careful — this steam contains lye.*

Thorough stirring is important because unmixed caustic soda beads will quickly fuse together to form a solid white mass on the bottom of the container. This fused lye can be dissolved by setting the container (covered, to avoid inhalation of lye fumes) in a pan of boiling water. The heat will eventually dissolve this mass into the rest of the soda-water solution.

➲ Mix the solution right before you heat the oils. By the time the oils have melted, the solution should have cooled down to the proper temperature: about 135 to 145°F (57–62°C).

3 Heat the Oils

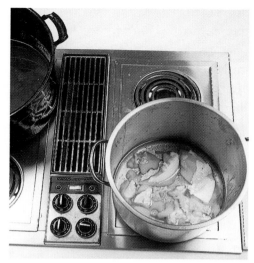

Weigh the fats and oils, then add them to the soap pot. **Melt over medium heat.** Continue heating until the temperature reaches 135 to 145°F (57–62°C).

 MIXING WITH A VARIABLE-SPEED DRILL MIXER

If you construct a variable-speed drill mixer, as outlined in chapter 7, place the mixer over the pot, turn the mixer on medium, and run the lye through the funnel. The mixture will trace more quickly than soap stirred by hand, but not as quickly as soap that's been run through a blender. Check the temperature occasionally. If it drops much below 135°F (57°C), gently warm the pot on medium-low heat.

4 Add Lye and Bring to a Trace

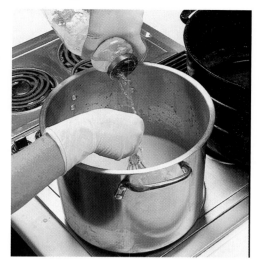

With your gloves and goggles on, begin adding the hot lye to the hot oils in a thin, slow stream. Stir steadily and continuously.

The lye solution and oils should both have a temperature range of 135 to 145°F (57–62°C). This temperature is substantially higher than the range used for cold-process soaps to accelerate saponification and help ensure a more neutral pH. If the temperature of the lye solution falls much below 135°F (57°C), set the container in a sink or pot filled with boiling hot water.

Soap made with the paste method must be stirred until it traces. Anything less spells failure.

After pouring all the lye into the oil, stir until the mixture thickens and "traces," which means that when a small amount of the soap is scooped up and drizzled over the mixture's surface, it leaves a trace or trail before sinking back in. Sometimes this is hard to detect unless the angle of light is just right. Tracing soap is the consistency of a light gravy or sauce; its color will also be whiter than when the lye and oil were first combined. Tracing can happen in as little as 3 minutes (when you are using a blender) or can take up to an hour (when you are stirring by hand). It depends upon the oils used and how quickly the mix is stirred. Don't try to shortcut on time — you must stir the soap until it's traced, otherwise the soap will separate.

If you are stirring the soap with anything besides a blender or food processor, check the temperature occasionally. If it drops much below 135°F (57°C) before tracing, place the pot over medium-low heat, and gently bring the temperature back up.

USING A BLENDER, STICK BLENDER, OR FOOD PROCESSOR

The fastest and easiest way to trace soap is with a blender, stick blender, or food processor. The procedure is as follows:

⇨ If using a blender or food processor, first stir the lye solution into the oils by hand, and mix for a minute to ensure a homogenous blend. (You'll want to do this in a lye-proof container other than the soap pot, since the blenderized soap will be emptied into the soap pot.) If using a stick blender, proceed directly to blending.

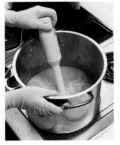

⇨ Pour enough of this mixture into the blender to fill the blender halfway up. If using a stick blender, keep blending until the mixture traces.

⇨ Mix the soap on low speed until it traces — it will be the consistency of a thin pudding. This should take about 20 to 30 seconds.

⇨ Empty it into the soap pot, then refill the blender with more oil-lye mix.

⇨ Repeat this process six or seven times, or until all the soap has run through the blender. Then briefly hand-stir the pot of blended soap to ensure a homogenous mix. Of course, if you're using a stick blender, you'll be able to complete the entire process in the pot at one time.

5 Cover the Soap and Allow It to Sit

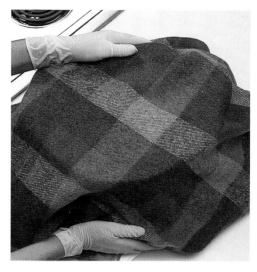

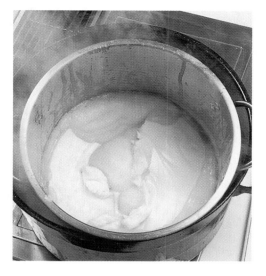

If you were making traditional opaque soap, color and fragrance would now be added to the tracing soap. The soap would then be poured into covered molds and allowed to harden. For transparent soap, however, you need to follow this procedure, which is known as the gel phase of soapmaking.

➲ **Place a lid over the pot, and wrap the bottom, sides, and top with a blanket or two.** The warmer the soap is kept, the more complete the saponification. Let the covered pot sit for an hour.

▼ Transparent soap must pass through the gel phase to achieve the proper consistency.

➲ **If you could watch the soap, you would first see it stiffen into a very thick white paste.** As saponification continues from the center of the pot outward, this white mass bulges slightly, then cracks to reveal a hot, amber-colored gel beneath. This transparent gel is the colloidal state, which all soap passes through before cooling. Soon all the soap is transparent and very hot — between 170 and 180°F (76–81°C). Successful transparent soap in large part depends on the soap passing through the gel phase — this is when the soap is neutralizing.

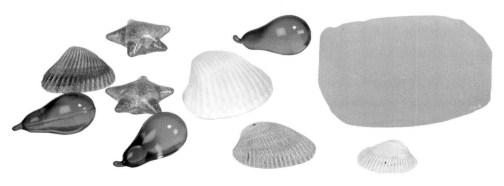

GELLING THE SOAP IN A DOUBLE BOILER

To hasten the gel time, create a double boiler. A 5-gallon canning pot is ideal. Pour 3 or 4 inches of water into the pot, and bring to a slow boil. Place a few spoons or knives on the bottom of the canning pot so that the soap pot has some water beneath it. Otherwise, the soap may scorch.

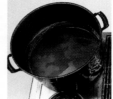

After the soap has traced, cover it with a lid and place it inside the canning pot. Keep the water at a gentle boil. Within 10 to 15 minutes, the soap will begin saponifying; a ring of softer translucent soap will appear around the circumference of the pot. Stir the soap for a minute, taking care to scrape the bottom. Cover again. In the next 10 minutes, stir briefly two or three times. Air trapped inside the soap mass may cause it to billow up, like a soufflé or rising bread dough. After two or three stir-rings, the air should be gone. The soap will then need only an occasional brief mixing.

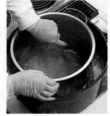

Neutralization should occur within an hour or a bit longer, but please test by dissolving a sample in water or by using phenolphthalein. You may then proceed with the addition of alcohol and glycerin.

Neutrality can be tested using phenolphthalein (pronounced fee-nol-THAL-een). This inexpensive chemical takes the guesswork out of pH testing. For instructions on its use, see page 42.

► If you carefully follow the outlined steps, your soap will come out perfect every time.

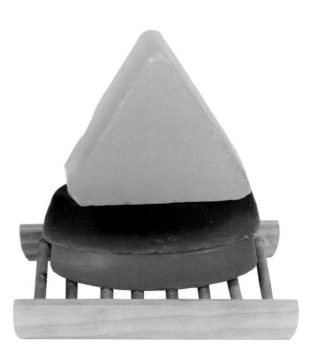

6 Stir and Recover

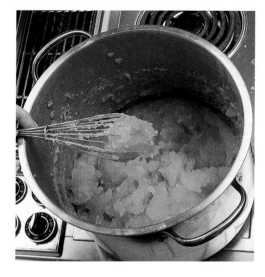

After stirring, cover the soap for another hour. Saponification is continuing, but eventually all the free alkalis and fatty acids will have reacted with each other, and saponification will slow. This slowing is signaled by a gradual drop in the temperature of the soap. The soap is now near neutral. If you want to test the soap for neutrality, take a small sample, drop it into a glass of distilled water, and stir. Neutral soap will easily dissolve. Another testing method involves the use of the chemical phenolphthalein. See page 42 for its use.

At the end of 1 hour, unwrap the soap. If it's still opaque and hasn't gelled, cover it back up until it does. The entire surface of the soap should be translucent, though there may be a thin white ring of cooler soap around the circumference of the pot.

Stir the gelled soap for a minute, taking special care to scrape away the cooler, harder soap from the sides and bottom of the pot. Incorporate this into the hotter mass at the center of the pot. At this point, any burns you might sustain won't be chemical, because the soap is neutralizing. Be more concerned about burns caused by the high temperature of the soap.

▶ Following safety precautions while making soap is of the utmost importance. Always wear protective gear and be prepared in case of an accident.

USING PHENOLPHTHALEIN

The chemical phenolphthalein has wide and oddly diverse uses. For the soapmaker, it functions as an acid-base indicator. I find it far more useful than pH strips.

Phenolphthalein can be purchased as either a colorless liquid or a powder that can be dissolved in water or alcohol. It turns pink or red in the presence of an alkali and remains clear in the presence of an acid. A pH of 7 (the value of water) is considered truly neutral. All pH values from 1 to 6.9 are acids, with 1 being the most acidic. From pH 7.1 up to pH 14, the values are increasingly alkaline. Soap is considered neutral, however, when it has a pH of about 9.5.

To use phenolphthalein, squeeze a drop directly onto a sample of soap after it's been through the gel stage. If a pink color appears, the soap contains excess caustic soda; the deeper the pink, the more the excess. Cover the soap and allow more time for neutralization. If it still tests pink after another half hour to an hour, add glycerin and alcohol, and proceed with mixing. Now correct the pH using the technique given on page 114. Add stearic acid a little at a time until the pink disappears.

If the phenolphthalein remains clear when dropped onto a sample of soap, the pH will be at 9.5 or below. The lower the pH, however, the higher the level of free fatty acids — which may manifest as cloudiness and greasiness in the finished soap. Correct by adding more lye solution (see page 114). Mix for 20 minutes, then test. Continue until the phenolphthalein registers the faintest shade of pink when dropped onto a sample.

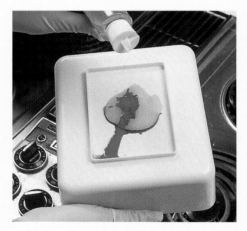

▲ If the phenolphthalein turns pink when dropped on a gelled sample, the soap is too alkaline.

7 Add Alcohol and Glycerin

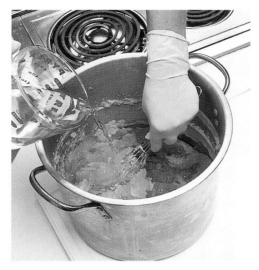

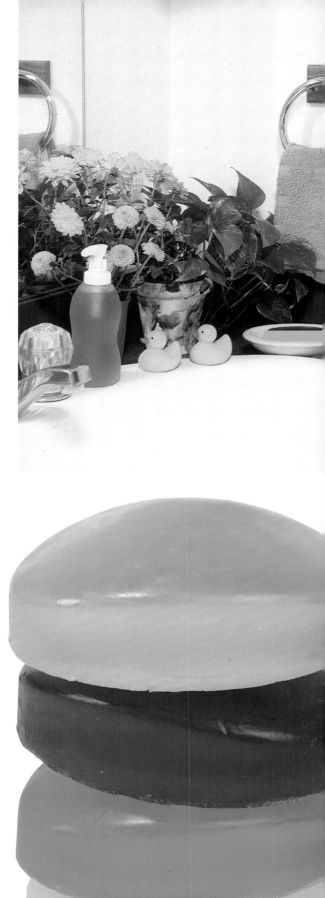

Before dissolving the soap in alcohol and glycerin, please take time to read through Safety Procedures for the Use of Alcohol (pages 32–33)!

Uncover the pot, and add the alcohol and glycerin. The soap is probably still in the gel state and is consequently quite warm. So stand back a bit when adding the alcohol. Alcoholic vapors will be created as the alcohol is heated by the soap. These vapors are heady. At the same time, the hot gel is being cooled by the solvents, and a portion of this gel now hardens into lumps of soap. Don't worry about these — they'll eventually dissolve.

▶ The addition of alcohol and glycerin will ensure that the opaque gelled soap will become transparent soap.

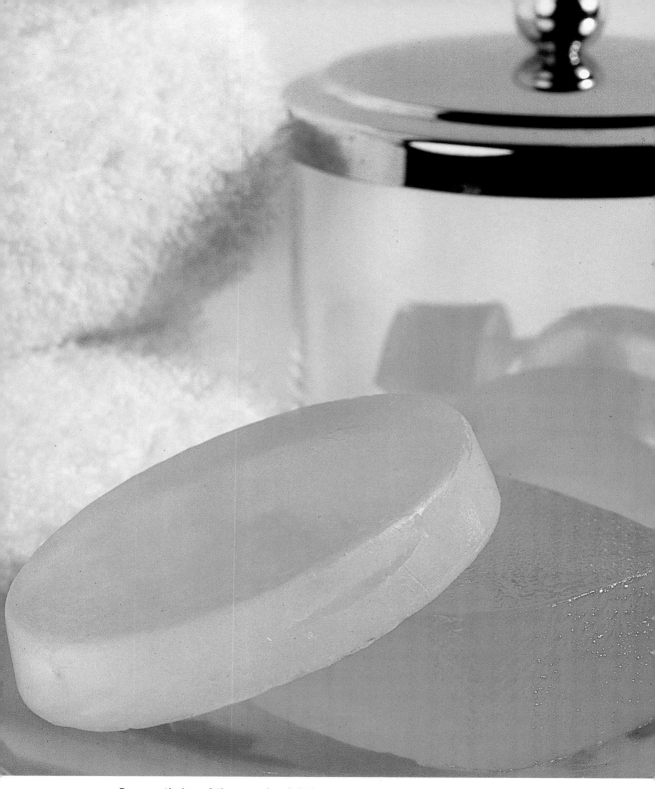

▲ **Proper stirring of the soap broth helps create a soap that is firm and easy to remove from its mold.**

8 Scrape the Bottom and Sides

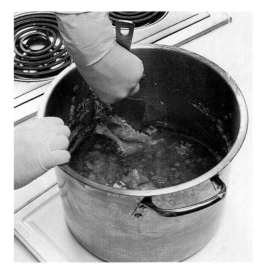

Now scrape all of the cooler, harder soap away from the bottom and sides of the pot, using a spoon or a spatula. Be sure to clean the bottom and sides thoroughly of any stubborn patches of sticking soap, particularly on the bottom of the pot. Soap left on the bottom will burn when the soap is reheated. Sticking soap can also flake off right before the finished broth is poured; you'll then have transparent bars containing flecks of undissolved soap.

Break up any large chunks with the whisk. Your soap won't be completely dissolved at this point, but it will dissolve when the broth is heated.

▶ A beautiful batch of see-through soap is easy to achieve with careful preparation.

If you're using a variable-speed drill mixer, the above procedure can't be done with the mixer. You must manually scrape the bottom and sides of the pot. Then the mixer can be placed over the pot and turned on. No plastic sheeting is necessary.

> Whisks are the best utensil to use when you are stirring by hand. They help break up the soap mass so that it dissolves completely in the alcohol.

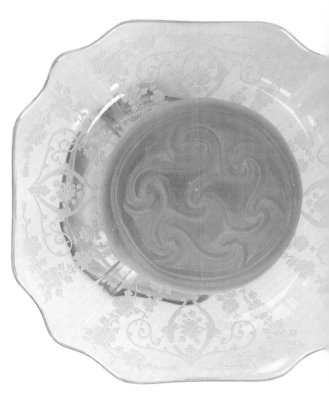

9 Make a Plastic "Tent"

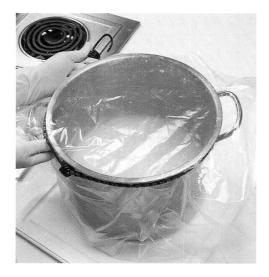

Now cut two pieces of 3 to 4 ml plastic sheeting, each piece large enough so that several inches overhang the entire circumference of the pot. **Secure the first piece of plastic tightly around the outer circumference of the top of the pot with rope or bungee cord;** the tighter the fit, the less evaporation.

➲ Pull gently on the outer edges of the plastic so that the excess is pulled underneath the rope or cord, creating a tight, drumheadlike plastic cap over the top of the pot. Repeat the process with the second sheet of plastic and the second rope or cord.

10 Heat Soap Solution

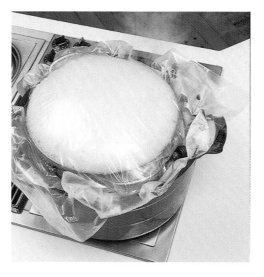

Place the covered pot into the double boiler bottom. Watch for the soap solution to come to a gentle boil, then adjust the heat to maintain the boil. Cook the soap for about 30 minutes. During this time, any undissolved soap should dissolve, since the boiling action of the liquid substitutes for the mechanical motion of hand-stirring. **The plastic tent will balloon as the air and steam expand, but don't get nervous;** the plastic is thick and won't rupture. If you still feel uneasy, remove the pot from the heat and pull the plastic under the rope or cords to tighten.

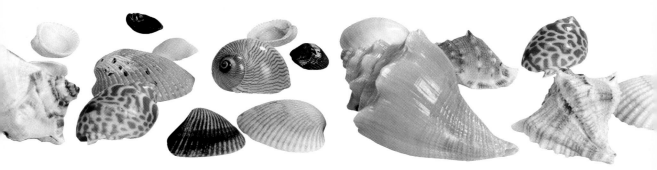

11 Add Sugar

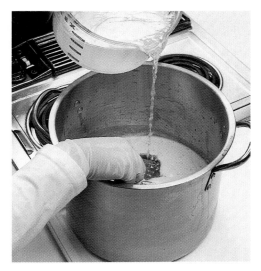

Sugar helps avoid the cloudy look that can so often happen in making transparent soap. Be sure to measure the sugar, though, as too much can cause the soap to "sweat."

↻ After 30 minutes of cooking, prepare a sugar solution. In a separate pan, bring the water portion of the sugar solution to a boil, then add the granulated sugar. Stir until completely dissolved. Cover the pan, and bring the sugar back up to a boil; let simmer for another 2 to 3 minutes. This will allow steam to wash off any undissolved sugar crystals adhering to the walls of the pot.

↻ **Unwrap the plastic tent, then stir the sugar solution into the soap broth.**

▶ **Transparent soap is as attractive as it is useful. Experiment with different colors and molds to create your own works of art.**

Before adding sugar solution, make sure all of the soap has dissolved. To do this, withdraw a small sample and pour it into a clear jar. Hold the jar up to the light; undissolved soap will appear as opaque specks floating in a clear amber solution. Cook longer to dissolve.

 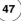

12 Test for Transparency

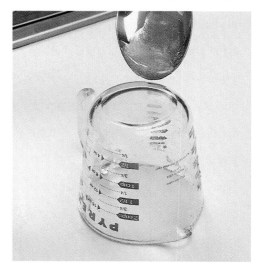

Ladle out a spoonful of the solution, and dribble it onto an inverted glass or bottle. (To hasten the hardening time, chill the glass in the freezer a few minutes before testing the soap.) The degree of transparency found in this hardened sample will be mirrored by the transparency of the entire batch after it has hardened in the molds.

Note: Sometimes the top surface of the hardened sample may be somewhat milky. Rinse the sample briefly in hot water to dissolve this skin. If the rest of the sample remains milky, please consult chapter 8, Troubleshooting.

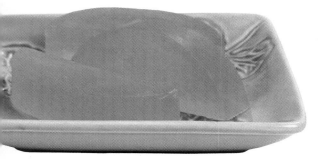

13 Settle the Soap

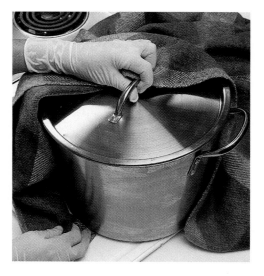

Whether your soap is right the first time or you've had to add a little extra of this or that, when a spoonful hardens and remains transparent, the soap can soon be poured. But first you'll need to exercise just a bit more patience. **Cover the pot for another 20 minutes, or until the temperature of the soap drops to 140°F (59°C).**

During this time the soap is cooling and settling. A cooler solution loses less alcohol to evaporation when the solution is poured into molds; cooler temperatures are also gentler on the fragrances. Settling the soap allows impurities in the broth to sink to the bottom and any air bubbles suspended in solution to rise to the surface. Foam caused by too much agitation usually disappears during settling, but if it doesn't, skim it off. Excess foam will harden. You can also fill a spray bottle with ethanol or isopropyl alcohol, then aim the spray at the foam. A few squirts will subdue even the most stubborn head of foam. *Be sure to avoid spraying the alcohol mist near gas flames.*

14 Add Dye and Fragrance

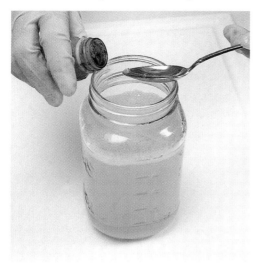

ENSURING TRANSPARENCY

As explained earlier, rapid cooling helps ensure transparency, so don't cover the molds or pour the soap into molds that are excessively deep. Your soap will harden in 1 to 6 hours. The speed with which it hardens depends on two things: the size of the mold and the formulation of the soap.

When the pot is uncovered this last time, the solution will have cooled down a bit. There will be a thin skin of hardening soap on the surface. A few stirs will dissolve this layer. If the skin resists melting, this means that the soap stock is too cool, so put the pot back on the stove, heat it, and stir for a minute or two until everything's dissolved. This skin won't ruin your soap, but if it isn't dissolved back into the solution it creates a blemish in the finished bar.

⊃ Now the soap is ready for the addition of the fragrance and dye unless you prefer a neutral bar. Color and fragrance are added to the liquid stock after it has settled for 15 or 20 minutes. **With the soap in the pot or a jar, pour a small amount of dye or fragrance onto a teaspoon; add it to the soap.** Stir to incorporate.

Coloring and fragrancing ideas are presented in detail in chapter 5.

▶ Choose bright dyes and strong fragrances to create soaps that leave a lasting impression.

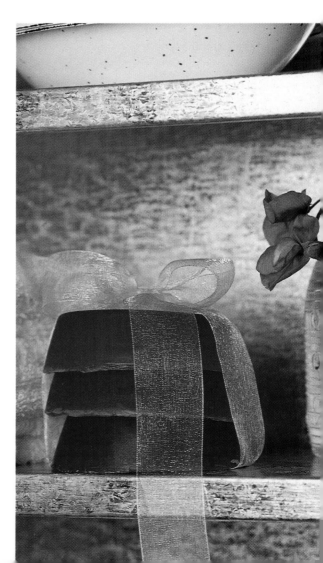

selecting a mold

What should a soapmaker look for when buying soap molds? Three things: strength, flexibility, and "draft."

Many types of plastic are suitable for soap molds, but whether you're pouring into Tupperware containers or into custom molds designed specifically for soapmaking, the plastic should have enough flexibility or "give" to release the soap. Thin plastic is always more flexible than thick plastic, but it is also weaker and less durable. Look for molds that strike a happy balance between strength and flexibility.

Draft is an equally important consideration. Soap poured into a rectangular cavity with 90-degree sides is removed from the mold with much more difficulty than a cavity tapered inward from base to top. This taper, called draft, is ideally an angle of 7 to 12 degrees. The more draft, the easier the release. As logical as that sounds, some molds on the market not only lack draft, but are actually narrower at the cavity's base than at its top.

Draft should be designed into the details of the mold as well. For example, if you buy a flower mold, all of the design elements of that mold from stem to petals need draft. Beware of molds with any undercuts, or notched designs. Undercutting may lend beauty and drama to a design, but it also prevents the soap from being removed from the mold.

Here are some other tips to keep in mind when using molds:

• Keep the soap on the double boiler as you dye and fragrance; cooling soap begins to harden before it reaches the molds.

• If your molds are made of clear plastic, check for air bubbles (cooked soap is more viscous than uncooked). These bubbles can be dislodged by gently tapping the mold on the counter top. If the soap seems too viscous, a few ounces of ethanol will help make it a bit easier to pour, although alcohol softens the soap's consistency.

• Transparent or melt-and-mold soaps usually unmold with great ease. If you encounter any difficulty, set the molds in warm water for a half a minute or so — the slight melting along the soap/plastic interface should do the trick.

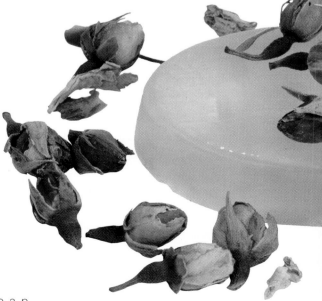

15 Mold

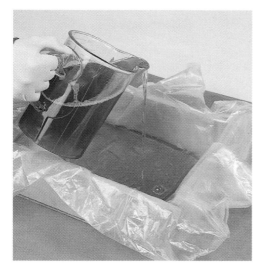

Place the molds on a level surface where they can sit undisturbed for several hours. Lay some newspaper under them in case of spillage. **Pour soap solution into mold.** Unless you're pouring into one large mold, you'll probably want to use a ladle or lipped measuring cup for filling smaller molds with the watery broth.

16 Let Harden

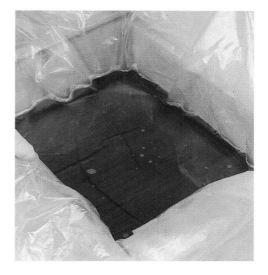

Before unmolding, make sure the soap is completely firm by pressing in the middle and feeling for any "give." Out of haste you might prematurely unmold the soap only to find that the inner core is still runny, like a chocolate with a liqueur filling. The soap would then need to be remelted and poured again. Once out of the molds, your soap will be transparent except for the top surface. This will appear a bit opaque and slightly pock-marked because of the tiny air bubbles that have risen out of solution and impressed themselves there.

17 Create a Finished Look

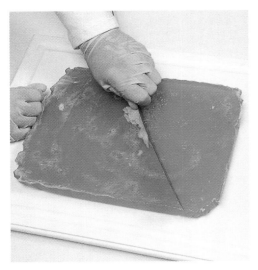

18 Cut into Bars

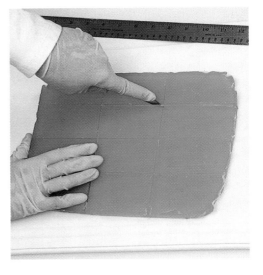

Take a knife blade or the edge of a ruler, and gently scrape off the blemishes. Alter the direction of your swipes so that no gouges begin developing in one particular spot.

You can further polish the soap by rubbing it with a soft cotton cloth or a sponge dipped in alcohol (either ethanol or isopropyl alcohol). The alcohol slightly dissolves the surface and gives the soap a more finished look.

To cut a large slab of soap into bars:

➲ First measure off the desired bar sizes with a ruler or a T-square.

➲ Gently score this grid into the top surface of the slab with a knife.

➲ After the slab is marked off, the bars can be cut with the knife or a pastry blade. A stiff paint-scraping blade works well, too. If these bars are too thick, turn them on their sides, and cut them to the desired thickness. Whether or not you've poured the soap into individual molds or into one large slab, the recipes in this book will yield between 40 and 50 average-sized bars.

◄ **Simple geometric shapes can be made easily with many different types of molds.**

19 Cure the Soap Bars

The bars need to be cured and hardened for 2 weeks. A warm, dry place is best, but don't get overenthusiastic and set them in a warm oven or a sunny window. If the air is too warm, they'll melt.

Line the bars up on an empty storage shelf or plywood covered with waxed paper. Eighteen-inch-square plastic greenhouse trays work beautifully; the open grillwork on the bottoms allows for air circulation underneath the bars as well as around the sides and tops. Whatever you use, just make sure to leave a little space between the bars for air circulation.

During the curing time, a skin forms on the bars. Water and alcohol begin evaporating out of the soap. Not only are your bars hardening, they're also becoming more transparent. This increased transparency is subtle but noticeable.

At the end of 2 weeks, check the bars. Are they still a little soft? If so, give them another week. If you're impatient, go ahead and start scrubbing.

▼ More elaborate molds are available through mail-order suppliers. See Resources for information.

When cutting and handling the bars, take care to avoid leaving fingerprints. The clear, sticky surface of the uncured soap reveals all. Latex or thin surgical gloves are helpful for avoiding these unsightly blemishes.

 ONE FINAL NOTE

If for some reason you're dissatisfied with your finished batch of hardened soap, the soap can be cut up and remelted over a double boiler.

If you do remelt the soap, it's best to do it within the first few days of the initial pour. Alcohol and water will be evaporating, and you run the risk of reduced transparency or stickiness if you wait too long.

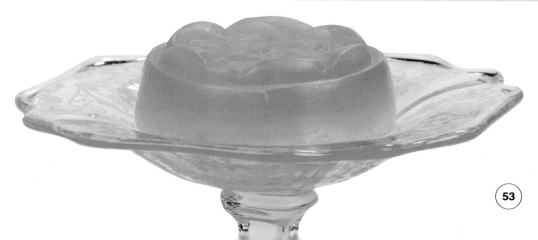

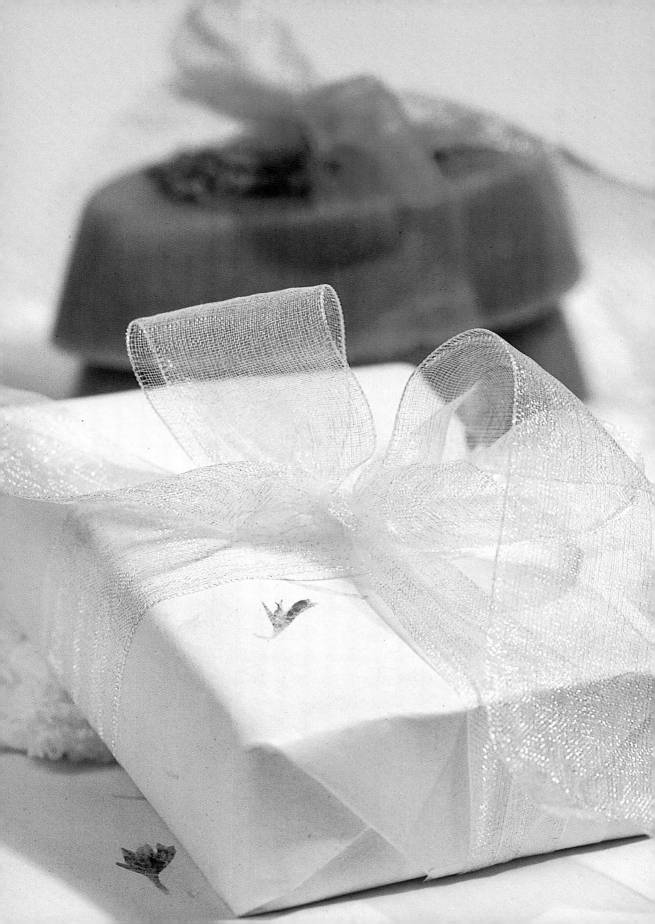

MOLDING COLD-PROCESS SOAPS

Cold-process opaque soaps vary in ease of release. In general, the more superfatted the soap or the higher the proportion of soft oils to hard, the more stubbornly the soap releases. In contrast, high percentages of palm oil or tallow produce firmer soaps that usually pop right out of the molds. For stubborn soap, set the molds in the freezer for an hour.

Another potential difficulty when pouring cold-process soaps into molds is heat loss. Soap needs a certain amount of heat to saponify properly and the greater the soap mass, the more internal heat is generated. Soap mold cavities, however, usually hold only 3 to 4 ounces of soap. That's a lot of surface area relative to the rather small mass of soap. Even when covered with several blankets, soap poured into molds at the standard 90 to 100°F (32–37°C) may not completely saponify.

Soft, grainy soap, or a crumbly "washed-out" appearance to part of the bar, is a sure sign of inadequate temperatures.

This problem can be solved in two ways. One way is to raise the pour temperature of your soap. Many cold-process soapmakers treat the 90–100°F (32–37°C) pour temperature as a commandment written in stone. Just remember that almost all soapmaking, for 20 centuries now, has been done at a full boil! Soap doesn't have to be treated with kid gloves. For small molds, pour your soap between 115–125°F (46–51°C).

In addition, hot processing avoids problems with poor soap curing. Use the double-boiler method outlined on page 46, cooking the soap for 1½ hours before pouring into molds. All cold-process formulations can be hot-processed; the only difference is that no solvents are added after the soap has neutralized.

◀ Handmade soap makes a welcome gift. Use creative packaging, such as colored paper and bows, for unique presentation.

the alcohol/lye method

The second method of making transparent soap is the alcohol/lye method. Alcohol is added to the oil/lye solution at the beginning of the soapmaking process rather than at the end. As a solvent, alcohol allows for much greater interaction between the oils and lye. The entire process will take about two hours. Another benefit of this method is that the soap requires virtually no stirring; it's accomplished by the mechanical action of boiling.

How to Do It

The procedure for the alcohol/lye method is as follows:

Step 1. Measure out the caustic soda and water. Mix and allow to cool until the temperature drops to 135 to 145°F (57 to 62°C). Heat the fats and oils and bring to 135 to 145°F (57 to 62°C). While the oils are warming, weigh out the alcohol portion of the recipe.

When the lye solution and the oils are approximately the same temperature, mix them together. Stir for a few minutes until a thin emulsion forms. Now add the alcohol.

Initially, the solution may form layers, with an oily slick on top. Stir for a couple minutes, then stop and watch for layering. If the oily layer persists, stir for a few minutes more. It shouldn't take more than 5 minutes to form a clear, homogenous solution.

Step 2. Prepare a plastic "cap" for the solution; this cap will prevent the alcohol from evaporating during the 2-hour cooking time. Cut out two large swatches of 3 to 4 ml plastic, large enough to not only cover the top of the soap pot but also enough to create 4 to 6 inches of excess drape around the pot's circumference. **Place one sheet of plastic over the top of the pot and secure it with a bungee cord.** Tighten the cord as much as possible; the tighter the cord, the smaller the amount of alcohol loss. Get rid of any slack in the plastic by pulling on the excess drape around the sides of the pot.

Secure the second sheet of plastic with a second bungee cord, using the same procedure. This second sheet of plastic substantially reduces evaporation.

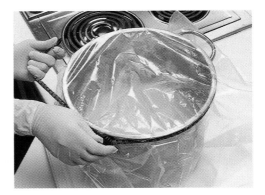

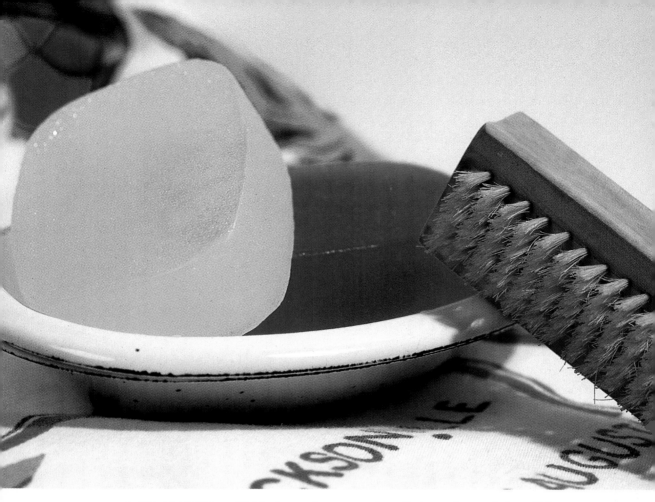

▲ **The alcohol/lye method also produces soap bars that are firm and clear. This technique works well for people who are familiar with handling alcohol and prefer not to wait long for the soap to gel.**

Step 3. Weigh the soap pot; this is its baseline weight. At the end of the 2-hour cooking time, you'll weigh the pot again to see how much alcohol has been lost through evaporation. If the plastic is tight, you may lose no more than 3 to 4 ounces.

Set the soap pot in the larger pot, which is filled with a few inches of gently boiling water. If the larger pot has a lid, use it — this will help conserve heat and keep your kitchen from steaming up.

Over the next few minutes, watch for the solution to begin boiling. The plastic will begin to puff up as the heat and steam build inside, but the plastic is too thick to rupture. When the solution breaks into a gentle boil, adjust the stove heat to maintain this boil. If the solution doesn't boil at all, the lye and oils may not neutralize properly. If the solution boils too rapidly, nothing is accomplished but a rapid loss of alcohol.

Once boiling, the soap solution needs about 2 hours of cooking time to neutralize. Check the plastic occasionally to be sure it isn't ballooning out from under the bungee cords. Tighten the plastic if needed.

Step 4. At the end of the 2 hours, weigh the soap pot before unwrapping the plastic. Compare this weight to the baseline weight. The difference between these two weights is the amount of alcohol lost. The loss of a few ounces might make little difference to the clarity of your finished soap; the loss of many ounces, however, will make a difference. But don't add alcohol just yet.

If you have phenolphthalein, dissolve a sample of soap in water and test. Does a light pink tinge appear? If so, the excess alkali can be neutralized by adding an ounce or two of melted stearic acid to the hot soap stock. Stir for a couple of minutes, and then test again.

Step 5. Now stir in the glycerin and sugar solution. Mix for a minute or so, then ladle a spoonful of soap onto the top of an inverted glass or jar. Allow to cool. Is the hardened sample clear or a bit cloudy? If it's cloudy, the problem is most likely due to insufficient alcohol. Add a few ounces of alcohol, and test again.

If the cloudiness persists after you've added enough alcohol to make up for what was lost through evaporation, the clouding is due to another problem — perhaps excess fatty acids. Consult Troubleshooting for help.

Step 6. Cover and settle the finished soap for 15 to 20 minutes. Your soap is ready for dyeing and fragrancing when a cooled sample hardens and remains clear.

▶ **If you'd rather experiment with molds, fragrances, and dyes than the actual cooking process, melt and mold soap is a great alternative.**

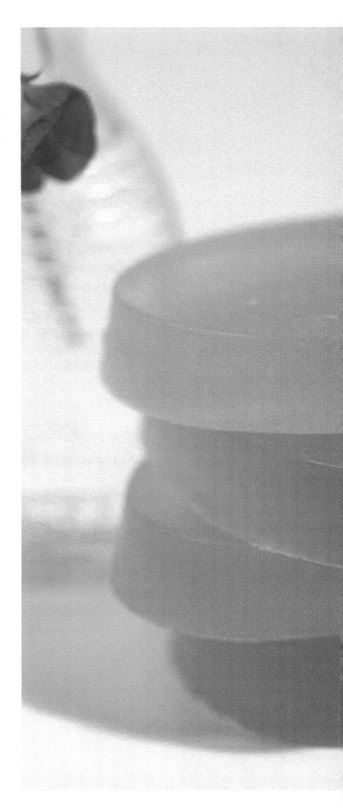

the melt and mold alternative

If you're wary of working with alcohol and lye or don't have the time to make transparent soap from scratch, soap-crafting with a meltable glycerin soap base is the next best thing and very easy. The soap base (available at crafts stores and through mail-order and the Internet) cuts like cheese and melts like butter. It hardens in a short time and is ready to use right away. Follow these steps, supplied by my fellow soapmaker Kaila Westerman, to learn the basics.

Cut and Melt the Soap

Cut off a piece of the soap base with a knife, and place it in a microwavable bowl or jar or a double boiler over hot water. Melt it completely, taking care to not let the soap boil over or get too hot. Overheated soap base can be brittle or have an unpleasant odor. Also, the hotter the soap base is when you pour it into the molds, the longer it takes to cool — and waiting for your soap to cool is the hardest step!

Add Color

You can use food coloring, but only for lighter shades. Too much food coloring results in a soap that will stain your hands or washcloth. You can also use small amounts of spices from your kitchen cupboard, such as turmeric or paprika. The preferred colorants are those manufactured specifically for soapcrafting. They are available through soap supply manufacturers. See Resources for more information.

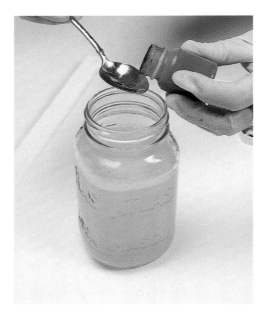

Add Fragrance

You may use your favorite perfume, or skin-safe fragrance and essential oils. Use about 1 to 3 teaspoons of fragrance per pound of soap. Keep in mind that the color of the fragrance will affect the color of the soap. For example, lemon essential oil will give your soap a yellow hue.

Other Additives

You can customize your soap with small amounts of skin-loving ingredients such as almond oil, aloe vera, and vitamin E. Generally, I recommend no more than 1 teaspoon of additive per pound of soap, as too much will make your soap feel like a less effective cleanser.

Pour into Molds

Many flexible plastic containers may be used as molds. Some great examples are candy molds, food storage containers, yogurt containers, and standard soap molds.

Use and Enjoy

Your soap is ready to use as soon as it hardens; no curing is necessary. If you want to sell your soap or give it away as a gift, you should first wrap it in clear plastic wrap to protect it from moisture.

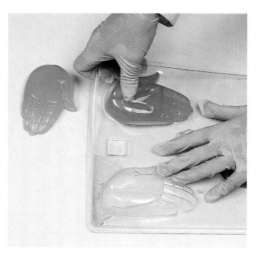

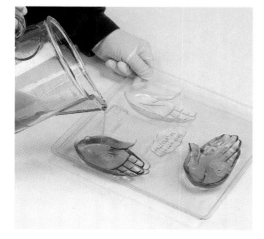

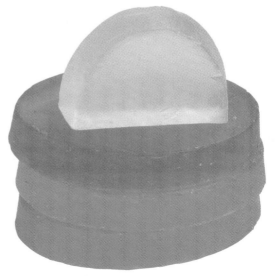

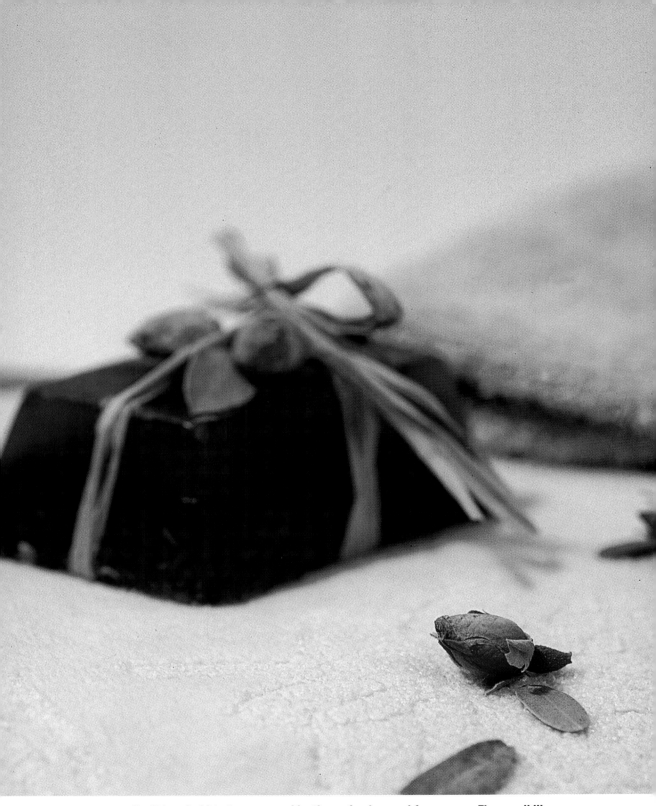

▲ Don't be afraid to try new combinations of colors and fragrances. The possibilities are almost endless.

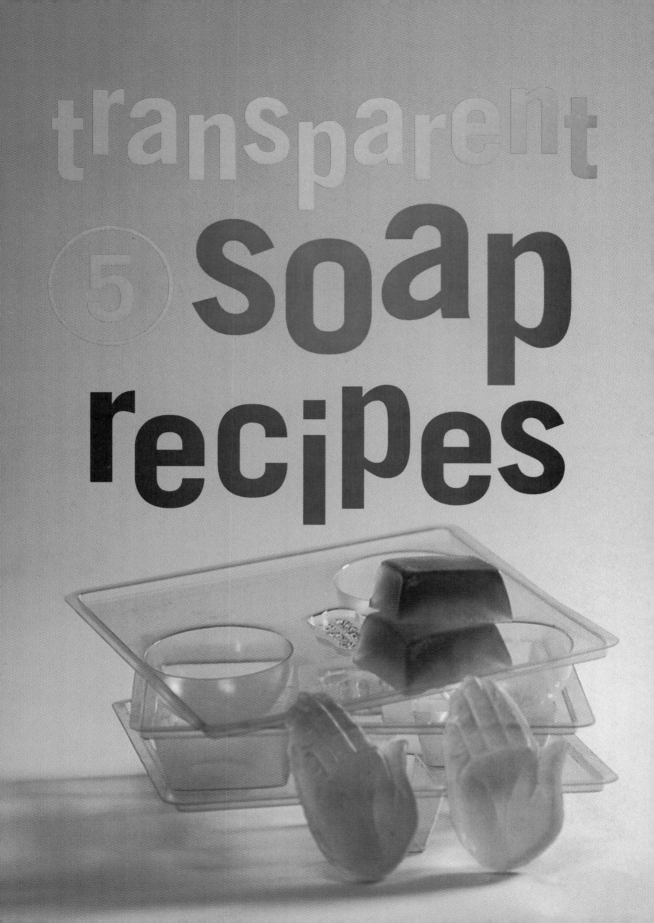

The following recipes all yield between 11 and 12 pounds (about 40 to 50 standard 4-ounce bars) of very clear transparent soap. The kinds of oils used, and the proportions of each in a given recipe, will produce bars of slightly varying hardness, color, and lather. Try a few different recipes, and keep a couple of bars from each batch for comparison.

Keep detailed notes. It's so easy to forget the details that make up your soapcrafting successes — or failures. Sometimes our "failures" become our greatest successes. For example, my Deep Amber Rosin Bars (see page 71) were a "mistake" — the result of mismeasured ingredients. But if I hadn't kept detailed notes, the mistake would have stayed a mistake.

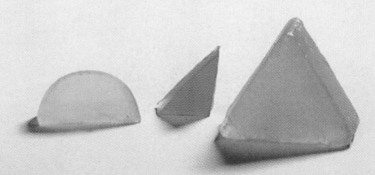

making substitutions

Each fat and oil used to produce a bar of soap has its own unique chemistry, which affects the soap's hardness, solubility, and lather. Here are some more specifics on which fats and oils can be substituted for others.

Substitutes for Palm and Tallow

Lard can be substituted for palm oil and tallow, but it produces a slightly softer bar of soap. For some of the following recipes (such as Basic Recipe 2 and Transparent Soap without Glycerin, which contain a high percentage of castor oil) the lard substitution might make the bars too soft. To compensate for this, subtract 3 or 4 ounces from the total weight of the lard, and use stearic acid in place of the missing ounces. Stearic acid will firm the soap. Melt the stearic acid separately, and add it after the other oils have traced. See the recipe for Transparent soap without Palm Oil, Tallow, or Lard for more details.

Substitutes for Castor Oil

Soft oils, such as canola, cottonseed, or olive oil, can be substituted for castor oil, but remember that castor oil acts as a solvent as well as a saponifiable oil. Therefore, soaps made with vegetable oils other than castor oil will have less transparency.

Substitutes for Ethanol

Isopropyl alcohol can be partially substituted for the more expensive ethanol. It is not as effective a solvent as ethanol; therefore, the transparency is inferior to that of soap made exclusively with ethanol. Isopropyl alcohol also possesses an odor that some people find offensive. Don't substitute isopropyl alcohol for all of the ethanol. Try a 25 to 35 percent substitution. When purchasing the isopropyl alcohol at your local drugstore, be aware that different concentrations are sold, some containing more water than others. A 99 percent solution is the one to buy.

Substitutes for Coconut Oil

Palm kernel oil can be used in place of coconut oil, but not as much caustic soda is necessary for saponification. If you wish to make this substitution, please consult Choosing Your Oils on page 72.

▼ Although using substitutions for fats, oils, and alcohol can affect the clarity of the soap, these batches of soap will have their own beauty and appeal.

 ALTERING QUANTITIES

Do you want to reduce or increase a recipe?

Changes in quantities sometimes adversely affect a formulation. See Formulating Opaque and Transparent Soap on page 72 for information that can help you avoid problems.

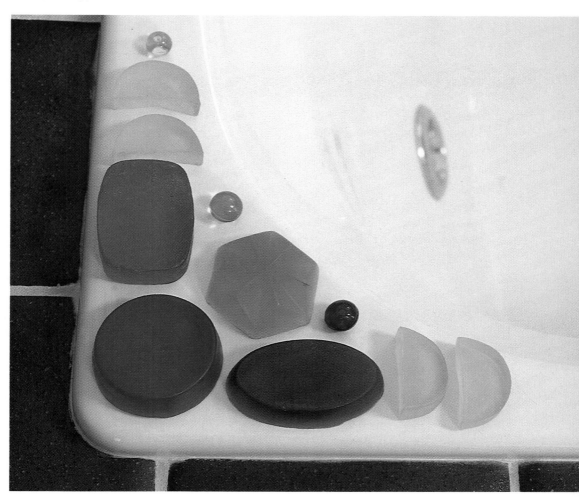

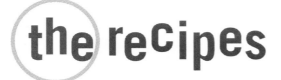

the recipes

These first three recipes are all very basic no-frills transparent soap formulations, but each differs slightly in the proportions of the basic oils. All yield very transparent soap with rich, creamy lather. You might want to make all three, setting aside bars from each batch for a comparison. This will familiarize you with the properties of the individual oils.

Before beginning, be sure to carefully read the step-by-step procedure outlined in chapter 4. Pay close attention to any relevant safety precautions.

Basic Recipe 1

Lye Solution
- 1 pound 9 ounces distilled or soft water
- 12 ounces caustic soda

Oil Blend
- 2 pounds 8 ounces palm oil, tallow, or lard
- 1 pound coconut oil
- 1 pound 9 ounces castor oil

Solvents
- 1 pound 12 ounces ethanol
- 8 ounces glycerin

Sugar Solution
- 15 ounces distilled or soft water
- 1 pound 4 ounces sugar

Basic Recipe 2

Lye Solution
- 1 pound 9 ounces distilled or soft water
- 12 ounces caustic soda

Oil Blend
- 1 pound 10 ounces palm oil, tallow, or lard
- 1 pound 11 ounces coconut oil
- 1 pound 10 ounces castor oil

Solvents
- 1 pound 13 ounces ethanol
- 15 ounces glycerin

Sugar Solution
- 13 ounces distilled or soft water
- 1 pound 2 ounces sugar

Basic Recipe 3

Lye Solution
 1 pound 9 ounces distilled or soft water
 12 ounces caustic soda

Oil Blend
 2 pounds 8 ounces palm oil, tallow, or lard
 1 pound 7 ounces coconut oil
 1 pound castor oil

Solvents
 1 pound 14 ounces ethanol
 1 pound 4 ounces glycerin

Sugar Solution
 13 ounces distilled or soft water
 1 pound 3 ounces sugar

▲ **Even the most basic transparent soap recipe yields spectacular results.**

Transparent Soap without Palm Oil, Tallow, or Lard

What works with this recipe is to warm up the coconut and castor oils in the soap pot, then add the lye solution. Stir until the mass begins to trace. This will happen fairly quickly because the lye is in excess. Now add the melted stearic acid. (Mix this by hand if you're using the variable-speed drill mixer — the stearic acid tends to clump, and the mixer can't blend it uniformly in the pot.) It will quickly thicken the coconut oil/castor oil soap stock, but the stock won't separate. If the mass appears a bit lumpy, try to whisk the lumps out as well as you can — but don't worry overmuch, because these lumps will be thoroughly incorporated when you uncover the soap in another hour and whisk it again. If you're using the alcohol/lye method, you'll avoid this problem since the soap immediately dissolves.

Other than this one simple difference, the rest of the procedures for this recipe are the same as those outlined in chapter 4.

MIXING STEARIC ACID AND LYE

This recipe uses stearic acid as a substitute for the palm oil, tallow, or lard. You'll need to mix the oils and the lye solution in a slightly different manner here. Since stearic is a pure fatty acid, it combines very rapidly with lye; within moments of pouring lye into an oil mix containing stearic acid, the soap can thicken so quickly that stirring becomes impossible. This thickening isn't the only problem. The accelerated reaction can separate the lye and the oil, curdling the soap. No amount of subsequent mixing can reunite them.

Lye Solution
 1 pound 11 ounces distilled or
   soft water
13 ounces caustic soda

Oil Blend
 1 pound stearic acid (melted and
   added separately)
 2 pounds 8 ounces coconut oil
 1 pound 10 ounces castor oil

Solvent
 1 pound 13 ounces ethanol
 1 pound glycerin

Sugar Solution
10 ounces distilled or soft water
 1 pound sugar

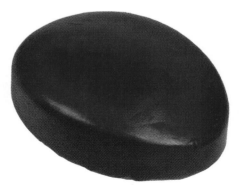

Copra Soap Transparent Bar

This is a recipe created exclusively for the transparent soap manufactured by my company, Copra Soap. The bar was designed to be mild, as transparent as other brands on the market, and firm enough to withstand the wear and tear of cross-country shipping.

Like the recipe on the facing page, this recipe contains stearic acid, so follow the same procedure given in the box at left.

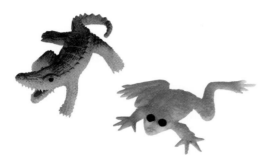

Lye Solution
- 1 pound 7 ounces distilled or soft water
- 11 ounces caustic soda

Oil Blend
- 1 pound 9 ounces palm oil, tallow, or lard
- 1 pound 9 ounces coconut oil
- 13 ounces castor oil
- 8 ounces stearic acid (melted and added separately)

Solvents
- 1 pound 13 ounces ethanol
- 1 pound glycerin

Sugar Solution
- 12 ounces distilled or soft water
- 1 pound 1 ounce sugar

Transparent Soap without Glycerin

The term *glycerin soap* has come to be synonymous with transparent soap, but as will be seen in the following recipe, glycerin isn't a crucial ingredient.

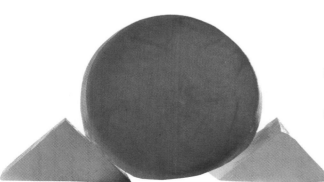

Lye Solution
- 1 pound 9 ounces distilled or soft water
- 12 ounces caustic soda

Oil Blend
- 1 pound 10 ounces palm oil, tallow, or lard
- 1 pound 10 ounces coconut oil
- 1 pound 10 ounces castor oil

Solvents
- 2 pounds ethanol

Sugar Solution
- 13 ounces distilled or soft water
- 1 pound 4 ounces sugar

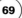

transparent soaps with rosin

Before we proceed to the next two recipes, a few paragraphs on rosin and its characteristics are necessary.

Rosin imparts wonderful qualities to transparent soap: a rich lather, an earthy aroma and color, and exceptional clarity. An excess of rosin in a formulation, however, creates soft mushy bars, or bars that dramatically effloresce within a day or two of pouring. Therefore, stearic acid is included in the following two rosin recipes to harden the soap and counteract this tendency.

Follow these instructions to avoid problems with your batch of rosin soap:

▶ Rosin has a very high melting point and also becomes sticky when heated, so mix it with the stearic acid (which also has a high melting point), and melt the two together on medium-low heat. Excessive temperatures will cause both the stearic acid and the rosin to darken.

▶ Stir occasionally to make sure the rosin dissolves. Since rosin is equally clear in both its solid and its liquid states, unmelted pieces can go unnoticed.

▶ After the stearic acid/rosin mixture has melted, add it to the melted palm oil/coconut oil blend.

Rosin has one more unexpected kink: when lye solution is added to a rosin/oil blend, the rosin causes the mix to rapidly thicken and curdle. Don't worry. Just proceed with the following steps:

▶ Whisk the lye into the rosin/oil blend as quickly and thoroughly as possible. The mass will appear quite lumpy.

▶ Cover the soap with blankets for 5 to 10 minutes.

▶ Uncover. The saponification rate is so accelerated by the rosin that the soap mass will already be gelling.

▶ Now the mixture will be a bit more manageable, so stir it for a minute or two. If the initial mixing wasn't enough to thoroughly homogenize the oil and lye, this second mixing should suffice.

▶ Now cover the mixture, and let it sit for the standard 2 hours.

Using the alcohol/lye method will help avoid problems with curdling, since the soap and rosin dissolve almost immediately in alcohol.

> **Rosin is distilled from the oleoresin of common pine trees.**

Deep Amber Rosin Bars

This recipe contains 1 pound of rosin — a lot of rosin. Make sure the rosin is well dissolved in the stearic acid before you add the mixture to the warm oil. The rosin imparts so much clarity to the soap that you'll notice a correspondingly smaller proportion of other solvents. The color of the finished bar is a rich nut-brown; the fragrance clean and earthy. You won't want to add any extra color or fragrance, since the bar stands on its own. This is one of my very favorite recipes.

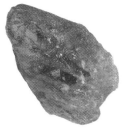

Lye Solution
   1 pound 9 ounces distilled or soft water
   12 ounces caustic soda

Oil Blend
   2 pounds 2 ounces palm oil, tallow, or lard
   1 pound 5 ounces coconut oil
   1 pound rosin
   9 ounces stearic acid

Solvents
   2 pounds ethanol
   14 ounces glycerin

Sugar Solution
   8 ounces distilled or soft water
   8 ounces sugar

Jurassic Soap With Rosin

Another beautiful bar, though a lighter amber — the color of pine sap. With its color and trace of piney fragrance, you can almost picture a 200-million-year-old insect embalmed within.

A great gift idea for kids: Drop a plastic insect into individual molds before pouring the soap.

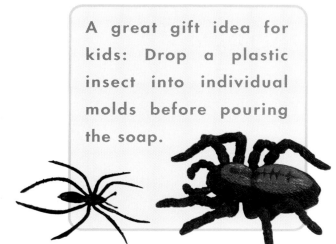

Lye Solution
   1 pound 9 ounces distilled or soft water
   12 ounces caustic soda

Oil Blend
   2 pounds 2 ounces palm oil, tallow, or lard
   1 pound 8 ounces coconut oil
   8 ounces castor oil
   8 ounces rosin
   6 ounces stearic acid

Solvents
   2 pounds ethanol
   12 ounces glycerin

Sugar Solution
   10 ounces distilled or soft water
   1 pound sugar

formulating opaque and transparent soap

These directions will give you all the basic information you need for formulating either opaque or transparent soap from a descriptive approach.

Soapmaking can be approached more scientifically using saponification numbers, iodine numbers, etc. This information can be found in soapmaking manuals in your local library.

Choosing Your Oils

First become familiar with the soapmaking properties of the basic oils. Chapter 2 and the following information should be enough to acquaint you with the oils. Then decide upon a blend — this is both an art and a matter of personal preference.

Many commercial opaque soaps are approximately 80 to 90 percent tallow or palm oil and 10 to 20 percent coconut oil. A formulation can be that simple.

The addition of a soft oil will give more of a cold-cream finish to soap, so a revised formulation could be 70 percent tallow or palm oil, 20 percent coconut oil, and 10 percent soft oil. Just remember that soap will lose firmness as larger percentages of soft oils are added.

More variables exist with transparent soap. The oils need to be blended with a little extra care, because blends that are suitable for opaque soap don't always work with transparent soap. For example, a high percentage of coconut oil is fine in opaque soap, but too large a percentage in transparent soap causes cloudiness. Then there are the solvents to consider. Solvents, as well as oils, have their own characteristics. A proper balance must also be struck between the solvents and the oil blend. Below are some general limits to keep in mind when you are blending oils. Guidelines for the solvents are given on page 75.

Palm oil or tallow. These oils form the base of both opaque and transparent soap. Either oil can account for between 30 and 75 percent of the total for the oil blend. I personally keep the percentages at about 50 to 60 percent.

Coconut oil. Too much coconut oil in a formulation clouds the transparency. Between 10 and 35 percent of the oil blend can consist of coconut oil or palm kernel oil.

Castor Oil. This oil imparts exceptional clarity, but an excess creates a soft, poor-lathering soap. Fifteen to 35 percent is a good range for castor oil. Remember that the more castor oil you use, the smaller the proportion of alcohol you'll need to dissolve the soap because of castor oil's solventlike properties.

Rosin. Like castor oil, rosin is both a solvent and a saponifiable oil. Rosin imparts even more clarity than castor oil, but it also creates more softness and stickiness. Keep the percentages a little lower than for castor oil — 5 to 20 percent of an oil blend. You might try adding stearic acid to counteract rosin's softening effect, especially when formulating with higher percentages of rosin. Too much sugar in a rosin soap causes efflorescence, so take care with sugar. This will be discussed in Solvents on page 75.

▼ **Once you've mastered soapmaking from a recipe, try formulating your own soaps from scratch. Formulating allows for better variety from batch to batch.**

The Caustic Soda Solution

After you decide on a blend, the next step is to calculate how much caustic soda is required to saponify the given amount of oil. The Dry Sodium Hydroxide Percentages chart below gives the percentage of dry soda (not solution) needed for each oil. Notice the range in percentages for each oil. Fatty acid content can vary according to how the oil is refined, how old the oil is (acid content tends to rise as oil grows older), and even the price of oil on the world market. When the price of coconut oil rises too high, this oil is often blended with less-expensive palm kernel oil, which greatly affects coconut oil's fatty acid content. When formulating, choose a middle percentage between the two extremes for each oil.

Assume you formulate a recipe by using 2 pounds palm oil, 2 pounds coconut oil, and 1¼ pounds castor oil. Refer to the chart. It takes approximately 14.3 percent dry caustic soda to saponify a given amount of palm oil. Convert the 2 pounds palm oil into ounces (32), and multiply by 0.143. You need 4.5 ounces caustic soda to neutralize the palm oil. Use the same calculations for the coconut oil and castor oil. Coconut oil requires 0.183 ounces caustic soda per 32 ounces oil, or 5.9 ounces. Multiply 0.13 times 20 ounces of castor oil for 2.6 ounces caustic soda. Add these three numbers up, and the total amount of caustic soda will be 13 ounces.

For the water portion of the soda solution, all the recipes in this book have been calculated on the basis of a fairly standard-strength lye solution: 32.5 percent caustic soda to 67.5 percent water. Dividing 67.5 by 32.5 equals 2.08. That's the constant you'll use for the soda/water solutions. If you multiply 13 ounces of dry caustic soda by 2.08, you'll need 27 ounces of water (or a total of 40 ounces lye solution).

Dry Sodium Hydroxide Percentages

These are the percentages of sodium hydroxide necessary to saponify common oils, fats, and fatty acids.

Fat, Oil, or Fatty Acid	Percentage
Castor Oil	12.8 to 13.2
Coconut Oil	17.9 to 18.8
Corn Oil	13.2 to 13.8
Cottonseed Oil	13.6 to 14
Lard	13.6 to 14
Oleic Acid	13.5 to 14
Olive Oil	13.5 to 14
Palm Kernel Oil	15.3 to 15.6
Palm Oil	14 to 14.6
Rosin	12.1 to 13.8
Soybean Oil	13.4 to 13.6
Stearic Acid	13.75 to 14.25
Tallow	13.8 to 14.3

Solvents

Soapmakers now need to calculate the proportions of alcohol, glycerin, and sugar solution for their transparent soaps.

Below are some general guidelines for these ingredients. Keep in mind that these numbers as well as those for the oils don't represent iron-clad rules. Straying a few percentage points in either direction won't ruin your soap. But these numbers do offer a good starting place and give some insight into the balance necessary for successful transparent soap.

Alcohol. This is the primary solvent for all transparent soap. Multiply the total weight of actual soap by 30 to 35 percent for the weight a formulation needs in alcohol. Actual soap is the weight of the oils and dry caustic soda. The water in the lye solution is counted as a solvent, not part of the actual soap. For example, if you have a formulation requiring 80 ounces of oil and 12 ounces of caustic soda beads, the weight of actual soap is 92 ounces; therefore, 92 x 0.30 or 0.35 = 28 to 32 ounces of alcohol necessary to dissolve the soap. Remember, the more castor oil or rosin in the oil blend, the less alcohol is necessary.

Water. Water should account for approximately 12 to 20 percent of the formulation's weight. This includes the water in both the lye and sugar solutions.

Glycerin. Excellent for transparency, but too much causes softness and sweating. Eight to 12 percent glycerin per total weight of the formulation is a good guideline. Glycerin can be replaced partially or completely by extra sugar solution.

Sugar. Similar to glycerin, but even better at producing transparency ounce per ounce. Too much causes softness, stickiness, and even efflorescence. Try to keep the total proportion of sugar (dry, not the total weight of the solution) at about 6 to 9 percent of the recipe. If you're formulating without glycerin, sugar can account for up to 13 to 14 percent of the total.

Transparent soap consists of approximately 50 to 60 percent actual soap to 40 to 50 percent solvent. When formulating a recipe, first calculate the oils and caustic soda proportions. From these numbers, find the weight of actual soap. Then take this number and calculate the recipe in two ways: one at 60 percent soap to 40 percent solvent, the other at 50 percent soap to 50 percent solvent.

Make the soap, then add the amount of solvents called for in the 40 percent formulation. After adding sugar and testing for transparency, evaluate the hardened sample. If it lacks a good transparency, refer to your 50/50 soap-to-solvent formulation. Using simple subtraction, calculate how much more of each solvent the 40 percent mixture will require to bring it up to the 50/50 mixture. Weigh each of the solvents, and begin adding them to the 60/40 solution a few ounces at a time, testing on glass after each addition. If a good transparency is achieved at 55 percent soap to 45 percent solvent, stop there. More is not better. More is softer. Then weigh what's left of each remaining solvent. Extrapolate from this figure just how much was added to the 40 percent solution. These additional ounces plus the numbers of the 40 percent solution become your recipe.

Confused? Let's apply these principles to the formulation from The Caustic Soda Solution: 2 pounds tallow or palm oil, 2 pounds coconut oil, 1 pound 4 ounces castor oil, and 13 ounces dry caustic soda. This totals 97 ounces actual soap. For the 40 percent solvent number, multiply 97 by 0.8, or 77 ounces of solvent. (Use 0.8 for all 40 percent solvent calculations.)

So if the transparency isn't satisfactory at 60/40, you have another 20 ounces of solvent to add before a 50/50 blend is created. These 20 ounces consist of an additional 5 ounces of alcohol, 5 ounces of glycerin, and 10 ounces of water. I usually withhold 3 or 4 ounces of the water just in case the transparency isn't quite right at 50/50. I then add a few ounces of extra sugar to this remaining water and try to get the proper clarity without having to add extra liquid.

I'm very conservative when formulating a recipe containing rosin, especially with the percentages of sugar. I start with sugar accounting for approximately 3 to 4 percent of the total. Soap without rosin is generally forgiving of excesses in sugar; soap containing larger percentages of rosin is not.

A final note if you want to increase or decrease any of the recipes in this book: I strongly recommend using the procedure outlined above for a 60/40 mix and a 50/50 mix. When doubling or tripling a recipe, I've occasionally noticed that less solvent is necessary. If you want to decrease a recipe, please use the double-boiler method outlined on page 40. A smaller mass of soap will generate less heat in the gel stage — this soap may not neutralize properly. The double-boiler method provides an external heat source to compensate for the loss of chemical heat.

▼ **With the correct balance of oils, solvents, and additives, you can make homemade soap that rivals any commercial brand.**

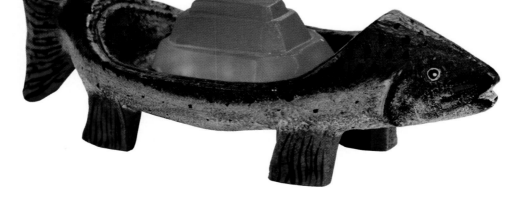

SAMPLE RECIPE CALCULATIONS

A recipe at 40 percent might look something like this:

ACTUAL SOAP

2 pounds palm oil
2 pounds coconut oil
1 pound 4 ounces castor oil
13 ounces caustic soda
_____
97 ounces actual soap

SOLVENTS

1 pound 11 ounces water (in lye solution)
1 pound 13 ounces alcohol (97 x 0.30)
1 pound glycerin
5 ounces water (in sugar solution)
_____
77 ounces solvents

97 ounces actual soap plus 77 ounces of solvent equals 174 ounces. For the amount of sugar you'll need, multiply 174 times 0.07 or 0.08. This equals approximately 13 ounces. Add this number to 174 ounces, and your total recipe will weigh 187 ounces. Of that, water accounts for 17 percent, glycerin for 8.5 percent, and sugar for 7 percent.

A recipe at 50 percent might look something like this (you'll need 97 ounces of solvents, which is 20 ounces more than the total solvents needed for the 60/40 formulation):

ACTUAL SOAP

2 pounds palm oil
2 pounds coconut oil
1 pound 4 ounces castor oil
13 ounces caustic soda
_____
97 ounces actual soap

SOLVENTS

1 pound 11 ounces water (in lye solution)
2 pounds 2 ounces alcohol (97 x 0.35)
1 pound 5 ounces glycerin
15 ounces water (in sugar solution)
_____
97 ounces solvents

Thus, 97 ounces soap plus 97 ounces solvent equals 194. Multiply 194 by 0.07 or 0.08 and you'll need approximately 1 pound of sugar. The total recipe now weighs 210 ounces. Of that, water accounts for 20 percent, glycerin for 10 percent, and sugar for about 7.5 percent.

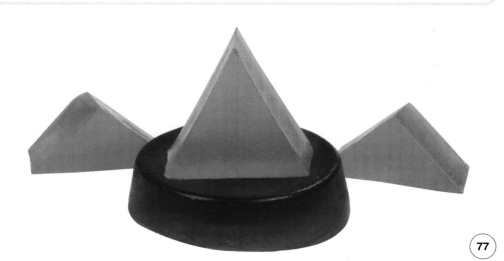

dyes
(6) &
fragrances

Fragrancing and coloring transparent soap is a delight. Stir in the dyes and watch the soap change into a liquid jewel — ruby red, topaz yellow, emerald green. Food coloring is all you need. Transparent soap can be fragranced with either natural or artificial fragrances, but no matter what you use, the fragrances remain true and fresh. The alcohol in the soap seems to act in the same manner as the alcohol base in a perfume — it "lifts" and intensifies the fragrances to such an extent that some soaps are almost edible.

Uncolored, unscented soap is beautiful too. Your bars will be a shade of amber and will have a light, clean smell. You might try dividing up the batch, pouring some plain soap directly into the molds, then dyeing and fragrancing the rest.

Color and fragrance are added to the liquid soap stock after it has settled for 15 to 20 minutes. The solution is a bit cooler after settling, which is better for fragrancing because the volatile fragrance oils will be less prone to evaporation or alteration by the heat.

dyes

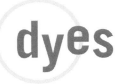

If you have ever made opaque cold-process soaps and have been frustrated by the skimpy palette of dyes available for coloring, you can unleash your creativity with transparent soap.

Many dyes take a battering from the high initial pH of cold-process soaps and are often altered beyond recognition. So unless soap dyes are special-ordered, the color range for cold-process soaps is pretty much limited to earth tones. Because of its neutrality, transparent soap can be tinted in either subtle earth tones or bright primary colors.

Food Coloring

Ordinary food coloring from the baking supply shelf of your local supermarket is all you need. Each set of food coloring contains red, green, yellow, and blue. The dyes come in either a liquid or a gel form. If you purchase the gel variety, don't add the gel directly to the soap stock. You can't control the color saturation as well because the clumps of dye will continue to dissolve over time. Squeeze some of the dye into a glass or a bowl, and add a couple of tablespoons of boiling water. Take a spoon or a fork, and stir until the clumps disappear.

Schilling sells a set of liquid dyes that come in 0.25-ounce squeeze bottles. Whether you're using liquid or gel food coloring, one set of colors is enough to tint several batches of soap. Be conservative with the dye. A little goes a long way.

Even though the soap is transparent, an oversaturation of color darkens the bar and consequently obscures the passage of light. The beautiful, gemlike quality of the transparency is then lost. To avoid this problem, start by adding just a few drops of dye to the stock. Pour some stock into a quart-size jar to a depth of 1". This will help you judge how the color will look in a finished bar. If you want a deeper color, add a few more drops of dye to the stock, and test again.

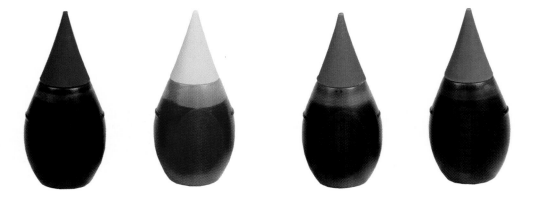

Blending Dyes to Make Custom Colors

If you've ever taken a basic design class, you are familiar with the color wheel and the methods of blending two colors to produce a third. Red and yellow create orange; red and green make a shade of brown; red and blue yield purple; yellow and blue produce green. Experiment a bit with mixing colors unless you're content with them the way they are. White cereal bowls work well for experimentation; the white background enables you to see just what the colors are without your having to dab them on paper.

Red, green, and yellow food dyes used in tinting soap remain stable and true in color. Blue is more problematic. It flattens and fades quickly — sometimes within a month or two. Exposure to direct sunlight hastens the fading. You might try dyeing just a small portion of the stock with blue (or derivatives of blue such as purple) so that the resulting soap can be used within a reasonable amount of time. The lack of a stable blue is the most lamentable shortcoming in food-grade dyes.

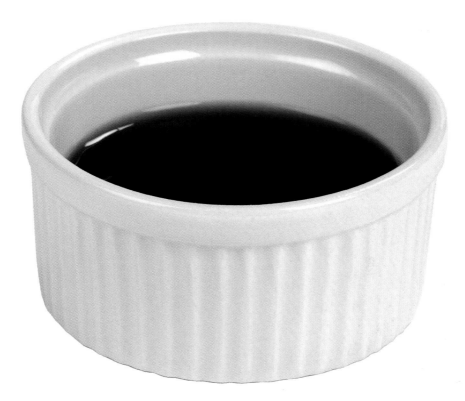

▲ **To make your own custom soap coloring, blend one or more hues of food coloring or soap dyes. Using a white bowl enables you to better view the resulting color.**

Natural Dyes

Besides the use of food coloring, you have several natural options:

• Pears, the original transparent soap, is tinted with rosin.

• Liquid chlorophyll comes in various shades of green, from a mossy hue to a brighter grass-green, and can be found in health food stores.

• Ground turmeric yields a rich golden yellow, and ground paprika produces an orange-red.

• Cocoa powder, curry, and a small amount of cayenne pepper are other possibilities.

Don't add any of these powders directly to the broth. Dissolve a few tablespoons of powder in a little water. Heat gently on the stove, then pour through very fine cheesecloth or an old nylon stocking. Tiny flecks of unstrained spice will be visible in your soap if you don't take care with straining — but perhaps speckles are the look you want.

Soap Dyes

There are limitations to food coloring. The lack of a stable blue is the most glaring, since blue is a primary color. Consequently, other desirable blue-based colors like purple and turquoise are also unstable and will fade with time. Aside from blue, colors such as ruby-red and magenta are also impossible to blend using the basic food-color palette. If you're frustrated by these shortcomings, try soap dyes — they're available in a much broader spectrum of colors. Suppliers are listed in Resources.

Note: Don't use fabric dyes to color transparent soap. These dyes are stabilized with salt. As mentioned earlier, mineral contamination can cloud the soap.

▼ **Natural dyes include ground spices and herbs, cocoa powder, rosin, and chlorophyll.**

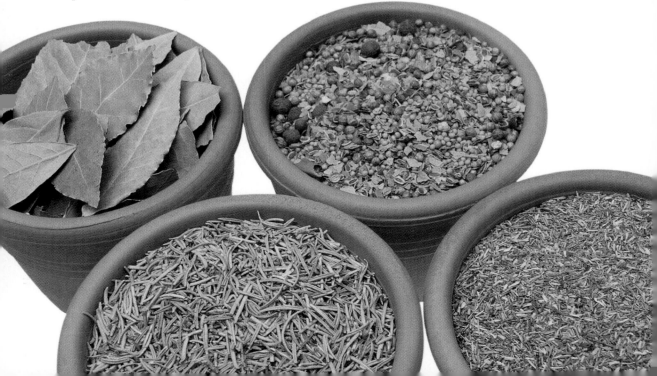

fragrances

Transparent soap is an excellent vehicle for fragrance. With opaque cold-process soap, the fragrance you smell in the bottle often flattens out or becomes almost unrecognizable in the finished bar.

Fragrances maintain their integrity in transparent soap, staying full and round over time. The lower alkalinity of transparent soap is a big plus; it could also be that the solvents help maintain the fragrance's character. At any rate, you won't have to second-guess the fragrances for transparent soap. What you smell is what you get.

> All fragrance notes, whether fruity, herbal-woodsy, spicy, or even musky, remain true to the bottled fragrance.

▶ Soap fragrances run the gamut from soothing florals to invigorating fruits.

Synthetic Fragrances

Some people have philosophical qualms about using synthetic fragrances. "They're not natural" and "they can cause allergic reactions" are the most common objections. However, synthetic fragrances aren't completely synthetic — they are usually blended with some true essential oils. And true essential oils can cause allergic reactions too.

Many delicious artificial fragrances are on the market now, such as passionfruit, dewberry, and piña colada; they make a perfect marriage with transparent soap. Most of these fruity notes go flat in a batch of cold-process soap; in transparent soap, you may find yourself wanting to take a bite out of the bar. This persistence is the reason why so many commercial transparent brands are so often fragranced with this particular family of scents. Other notes work just as well in transparent soaps: musks, spices, herbal-woodsy. (In Resources, you'll find essential oil and fragrance oil suppliers.)

Most commercial soaps are scented at 1 percent — that is, for every 100 ounces of soap stock, 1 ounce of fragrance is added. The recipes in this book all yield approximately 11 to 12 pounds, or about 170 to 190 ounces of soap; therefore, you'll want to add about 2 ounces, or 4 tablespoons, of fragrance. This is also a matter of personal taste. You may want to start with a bit less as an experiment.

Transparent soaps have another advantage over cold-process soaps: artificial fragrances don't cause the soap to thicken and "seize" in the pot before you have time to frantically pour it into the molds. If you have made cold-process soaps and have had this experience, you know just how horrible and hair-raising it is to watch all your expense and labor turn into an ugly lump in a matter of seconds. Cold-process soap contains a high percentage of unsaponified fatty acids and alkali before it's poured into molds. The solvents in artificial fragrances produce a larger "interface" between the acids and alkali, dramatically accelerating saponification. You can relax and take your time with the transparent soap. The oils and lye have completely reacted by the time the fragrance is added; the solvents in these fragrances can even impart a little more transparency to the soap.

> You can even try adding some of your favorite perfume to your transparent soaps.

Pure Essential Oils

Pure essential oils are extracted from plant materials using steam distillation or mechanical expression. It's a marvel that the wood, leaves, flowers, and fruits of plants can produce such a wonderful elixir.

There's much romance to essential oils. For instance, rose oil was mentioned in many ancient texts centuries before Christ, but this rose oil was probably not a true distillation from the flowers. Petals of roses were macerated, or soaked, in hot fats until the fragrance was infused into the fat. Legend has it that the first true rose oil was discovered by the wife of the Mogul emperor Jehangir in India.

The canals surrounding the emperor's palace gardens were filled with rose water, and one hot summer's day as his wife lazily drifted on the canals in her pleasure boat, she noticed an oily sheen floating on the surface of the water. She ordered that this oil be collected, and she named the highly aromatic substance Atr-i-Jehangiri.

Commercial perfumes are an orchestration of as many as 30 or 40 different oils in an alcohol base. Oils of "high," "medium," and "low" notes are blended for an overall effect, which changes with time, just as a fine glass of wine produces many flavors and sensations after it's been swallowed.

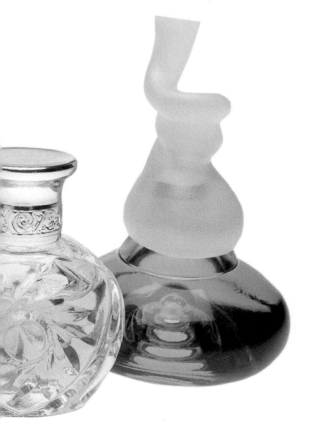

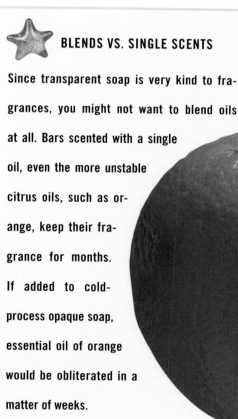

⭐ **BLENDS VS. SINGLE SCENTS**

Since transparent soap is very kind to fragrances, you might not want to blend oils at all. Bars scented with a single oil, even the more unstable citrus oils, such as orange, keep their fragrance for months. If added to cold-process opaque soap, essential oil of orange would be obliterated in a matter of weeks.

High notes are created by using more volatile oils with a high evaporation rate; citrus oils such as lemon, lime, and orange are especially volatile. The high notes are the first thing you smell in a perfume. They don't persist, however, and perfume changes character over time because the middle and low notes are emerging. These notes are composed of oils with lower volatility — that is, slower evaporation rates. Musk, patchouli, oakmoss, vanilla resin, and clary sage all have lower notes and actually act as fixatives for the fragrances of both soaps and perfumes.

You may want to create your own fragrances. There are books in print specific to perfumery; in fact, one such book gives the formulations for all the designer perfumes. Visit your local library. If you do start experimenting, use an eyedropper and test everything in small quantities before committing yourself to larger quantities. Always write everything down.

▼ **When it comes to fragrance blends, you should never feel limited to the recipes presented here. The only rule in soap fragrancing is to have fun!**

SAFETY WARNING ON ESSENTIAL OILS

Essential oils are highly concentrated and powerful. Many may burn skin if applied undiluted. Be sure to wear gloves when working with the oils, and mix well into your soap solution.

fragrance formulas

Below is a variety of fragrance formulations using pure essential oils. Each formula makes enough fragrance to scent one 12-pound batch of soap. Before investing in such large quantities of essential oil, you might want to experiment to find out just how a particular blend will smell. Using an eyedropper, make 1 drop equivalent to 1 teaspoon.

That way you won't use all of that expensive essential oil only to find out you really don't like the scent. Squeeze a drop of the blend onto a sheet of paper, and let it sit for a few minutes to allow the fragrance to change. Testing a few of these recipes by the dropperful will also give you a little more feel for perfumery.

White Lavender

- 6 teaspoons lavender essential oil
- 5 teaspoons geranium essential oil
- 3 teaspoons clove essential oil

Elderflower

- 6 teaspoons bergamot essential oil
- 3 teaspoons thyme essential oil
- 3 teaspoons peppermint essential oil
- 3 teaspoons lavender essential oil

Millefleur

- 8 teaspoons orange essential oil
- 3 teaspoons nutmeg essential oil
- 2 teaspoons clove essential oil
- 1 teaspoon lavender essential oil

▼ **Lavender is a time-honored fragrance used in many scent blends. The essential oil also has healing properties for the skin.**

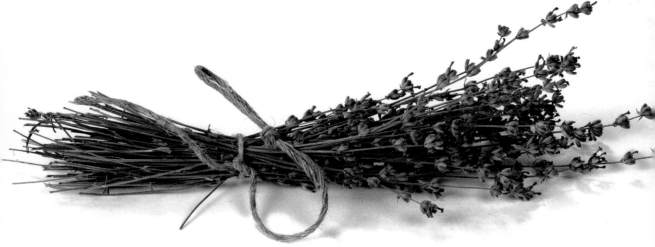

Brown Windsor

5 teaspoons clove essential oil
4 teaspoons nutmeg essential oil
3 teaspoons cassia essential oil
2 teaspoons caraway essential oil

White Windsor

4 teaspoons lavender essential oil
4 teaspoons bergamot essential oil
2 teaspoons thyme essential oil
2 teaspoons geranium essential oil
2 teaspoons clove essential oil

Rose

5 teaspoons bergamot essential oil
3 teaspoons rose or geranium
  essential oil
3 teaspoons sandalwood essential oil
2 teaspoons rosewood essential oil
1 teaspoon cedarwood essential oil

Almond

7 teaspoons bitter almond essential oil
7 teaspoons bergamot essential oil

Earth

5 teaspoons clary sage essential oil
3 teaspoons bergamot essential oil
2 teaspoons thyme essential oil
2 teaspoons sandalwood essential oil
2 teaspoons clove essential oil

Spanish Bouquet

4 teaspoons bergamot essential oil
4 teaspoons orange essential oil
2 teaspoons petitgrain essential oil
2 teaspoons sandalwood essential oil
1 teaspoon lavender essential oil
1 teaspoon patchouli essential oil

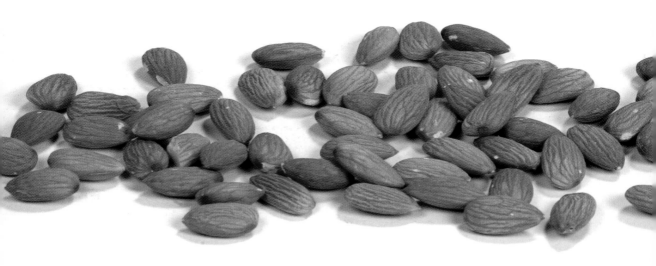

Lemon

7 teaspoons lemon essential oil
3 teaspoons bergamot essential oil
3 teaspoons lemongrass essential oil
1 teaspoon clove essential oil

Patchouli

4 teaspoons rosewood essential oil
3 teaspoons patchouli essential oil
3 teaspoons geranium essential oil
2 teaspoons cedarwood essential oil
2 teaspoons sassafras essential oil

North Woods

3 teaspoons spruce essential oil
3 teaspoons elemi essential oil
3 teaspoons rosewood essential oil
2 teaspoons vetiver essential oil
2 teaspoons bergamot essential oil
1 teaspoon cedarwood essential oil

▶ Molded soaps can be combined with an unusual dish to create a unique look for your bathroom.

▼ Flowers, spices, fruits, nuts — anything goes in soap fragrancing!

Bay Lime

6 teaspoons lime essential oil
2 teaspoons cedarwood essential oil
2 teaspoons cassia essential oil
1 teaspoon petitgrain essential oil
1 teaspoon lavender essential oil
1 teaspoon anise essential oil
1 teaspoon bay essential oil

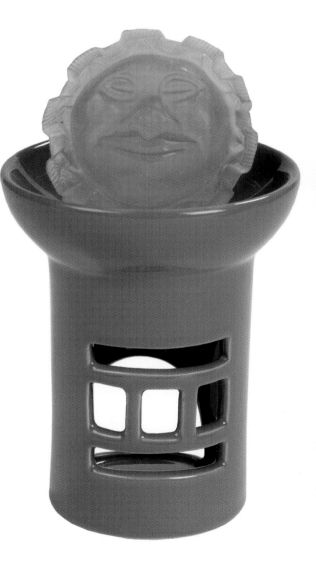

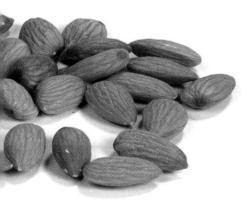

Honey

5   teaspoons lemon essential oil
4   teaspoons vanilla essential oil
2   teaspoons almond essential oil
2   teaspoons clary sage essential oil
1   teaspoon sassafras essential oil

Eau de Cologne

4   teaspoons bergamot essential oil
3   teaspoons orange essential oil
3   teaspoons lemon essential oil
2   teaspoons lavender essential oil
1   teaspoon bay essential oil
1   teaspoon rosemary essential oil

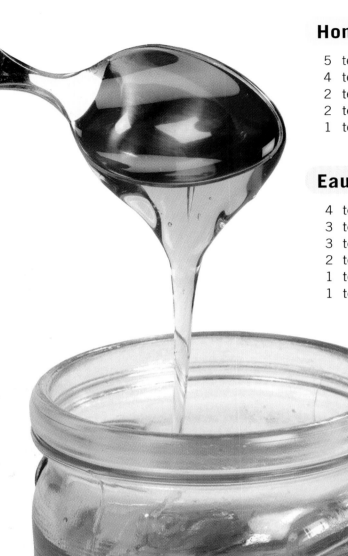

▲ Simulate the fragrance of real honey by combining essential oils (see above).

▶ Display your soaps in dishes, on bathtub ledges, or in the shower with your best spa sponges and brushes.

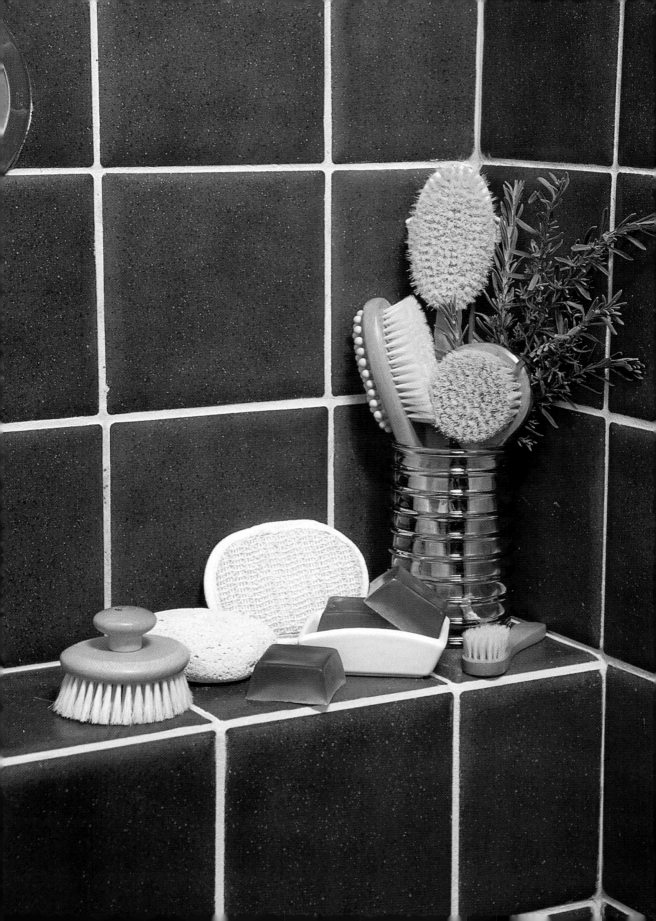

labor-
⑦ saving
tools

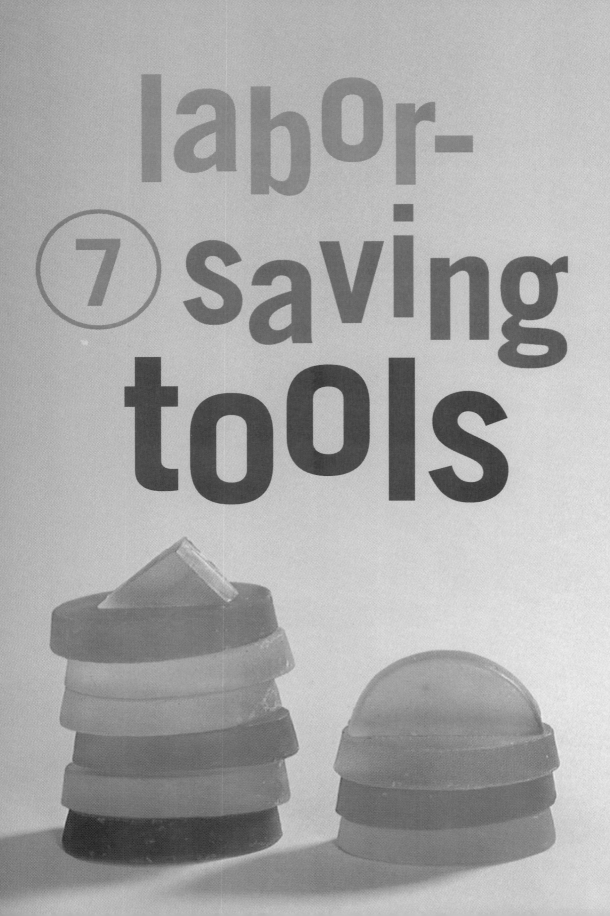

I f you're content with manually mixing your soap and hand-carving the bars, you don't need to bother with this chapter. But if you make soap — either opaque or transparent — more regularly and want to eliminate some of the labor of hand-stirring, and/or you want bars with crisp, wire-cut edges, read on. With a minimal investment of time and money, you can create a few tools that take a bit of the "hand" out of handmade.

This information may be of particular interest to small soapmaking businesses that make larger batches on a regular basis. These businesses often end up spending undue time on production, time that could be better spent on marketing or sales. Why spend an hour hand-cutting a 20-pound block of soap or hand-stirring a batch that just won't mix properly when these simple tools can cut the job to less than half the time?

adjustable-wire bar cutter

The light, portable cutter shown here will cost very little for materials and will take just a couple of hours to construct.

It's designed to cut a 12" x 12" x 2" block of soap into any conceivable square or rectangular shape you wish to create. Professional soapmakers have more elaborate cutters with stationary wires, but for the home hobbyist, nothing could be more simple and versatile than this adjustable cutter. You can also take the basic concept and create your own variation.

WHAT YOU'LL NEED

MATERIALS

- Two 2" x 4" x 28" boards
- Two 2" x 4" x 8" boards
- Two 2" x 4" x 3" boards
- One 1" x 2" x 28" board
- Two 1" x 2" x 20" boards
- Two 14" x 17" x ½" pieces of plywood
- Two 14" x 17" pieces of Formica or smooth linoleum (you should be able to find inexpensive scraps in the seconds bin of a flooring supply store)

HARDWARE

- Twenty-four 1½" and 24 2½" wood screws
- One ⅜" wide x 2" long hex-head carriage bolt
- Contact cement
- Medium-gauge guitar wire or 20- to 22-gauge music wire (sometimes called piano wire; see page 96)

TOOLS

- Drill
- Utility knife
- Hand or circular saw
- Socket wrench or crescent wrench

Assembling the Cutter

Step 1: Apply the two sheets of Formica or linoleum to the two pieces of plywood with contact cement. (*Note:* You don't need a special cutter for the formica — a utility knife will do. Hold a ruler or T-square on the line you want to cut, and gently but firmly score it several times with a utility knife. It will then snap along the line with gentle pressure.) Allow the adhesive 15 to 20 minutes of setting time before proceeding to the next step.

Step 2: With a few 1½" screws, attach the two pieces of plywood (Formica side up) to the two 28" two-by-fours. Leave a small gap between the two sheets — this will be the channel through which your adjustable cutting wire can slide. Countersink the screws so their heads aren't sticking up above the Formica surface. Otherwise, the heads can slightly gouge the soap as it slides across the top.

Step 3: Using a few 1½" screws, attach the strip of 1" x 2" x 28" wood to the Formica top. This is the guide edge for the block of soap as it is pushed through. Leave a ¾" margin between the guide and the edge of the Formica.

Step 4: Prepare the carriage bolt. Drill a hole through the shaft of the bolt, about ½" down from the top. Mount the bolt in a vise, and use a ⅛" or 3/32" drill bit; it takes just a few minutes to bore through the shaft. If you know someone who has a drill press or works in a machine shop, you might have him or her do it.

This bolt will function exactly like a tuner on a guitar or piano. Later, the cutting wire will be threaded through the hole in the bolt, and the bolt will then be tightened into a wooden block.

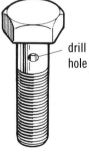

drill hole

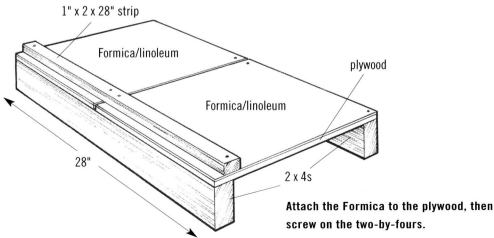

1" x 2 x 28" strip

Formica/linoleum

Formica/linoleum

plywood

28"

2 x 4s

Attach the Formica to the plywood, then screw on the two-by-fours.

Step 5: Take one of the 3" two-by-fours and drill a ¼" hole through the entire depth of the block. This is the channel for the carriage bolt, but since it's a bit smaller than the bolt, you might need to tap the bolt with a hammer to get it started in the hole. A snug fit is important, because pressure from the soap as it's pressed against the wire can unwind the bolt. The wire then loses its tension. The best way to achieve a snug fit is to follow this procedure:

⮑ Using a crescent wrench or socket wrench, tighten the bolt 1" into the wood.

⮑ With a smaller bit — ¹⁄₁₆" or so — drill another hole completely through the block ½" from the bolt.

⮑ Now take the other 3" two-by-four and drill a ¹⁄₁₆" hole through that too, about ¼" from the edge of the block. Partially sink a 1" wood screw into the middle of the block.

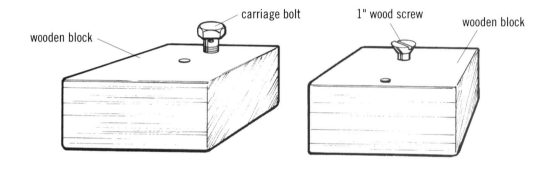

wooden block · carriage bolt · 1" wood screw · wooden block

 CHOOSING THE RIGHT WIRE

A medium-gauge guitar wire works well — you want to avoid a wire that's too fine, as it might snap as the soap is being pushed through. An overly thick wire will offer too much resistance to the soap. Buy one or two extra backup wires in case of breakage. Or you can get what's called music wire. This comes in a quarter-pound or half-pound roll and is much more economical than guitar wire. It's also more difficult to find. Try calling a piano tuner or rebuilder in your town — they might special order it or sell you some of their own. If not, contact the suppliers listed in Resources. A 20- or 22-gauge music wire is ideal for cutting.

Step 6: Screw or nail the two 8" two-by-fours onto the sides of the cutter. Make certain that the middle of each block is aligned with the groove between the two sheets of plywood.

Step 7: To the tops of these 8" two-by-fours, screw down the two 20" one-by-twos side by side, leaving a slight gap between them. This gap should line up with the groove between the sheets of plywood below.

Step 8: Thread the guitar wire or a 2-foot length of music wire through the hole in the carriage bolt. (The bolt should be tightened into the 3" block). Loop the end of the music wire once around the bolt, and tie a knot. You might have to use pliers to do this. Clip off the excess wire. If you're using guitar wire, run the length of the wire through the bolt until the metallic knob at the wire's other end hits the bolt. The knob is enough to secure the guitar wire — you don't need any knots.

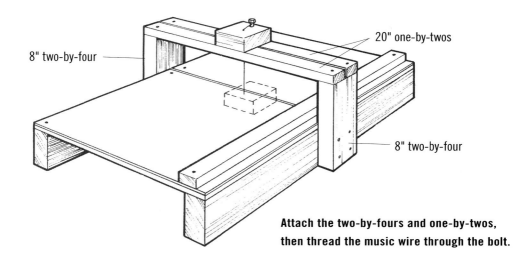

8" two-by-four

20" one-by-twos

8" two-by-four

Attach the two-by-fours and one-by-twos, then thread the music wire through the bolt.

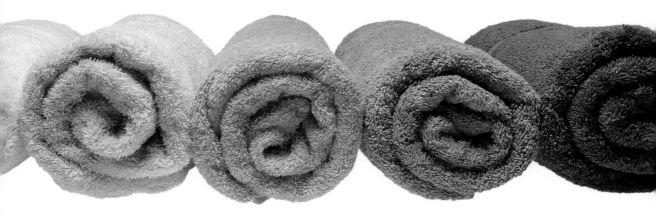

Step 9: Feed the free end of the wire through the ¹⁄₁₆" hole next to the bolt. Now set this block of wood on top of the two one-by-twos that form the "bridge" across the cutter. Pass the wire through the gap in the bridge, then on down into the narrow channel running the width of the Formica top. The wire should now be sticking out through the bottom of the cutter.

Step 10: Flip the cutter over. Thread the wire through the other 3" block, starting on the side without the wood screw. Pull the wire taut, wind it a few times around the screw head, and tie a knot. Sink the rest of the screw into the wood. This will secure the wire to the bottom block. Clip off the excess wire. Now, flip the cutter right side up.

Step 11: Tighten the wire by turning the carriage bolt with a socket wrench or crescent wrench. (Make sure you twist clockwise so the bolt sinks deeper into the wood. You don't want to be tightening the wire at the same time you're unscrewing the bolt from the block). The hex-head bolt functions in the same manner as a tuner on a stringed instrument. Don't tighten it too much — wire with too much tension tends to snap under the pressure of the soap. Make it tight, but not too tight. Attaining the right tension is a matter of a little experimentation. The tightened wire should hold the 3" block of wood underneath the cutter snug against the plywood.

Your cutter is done!

▼ Specially crafted tools make the task of cutting your soap a great deal easier.

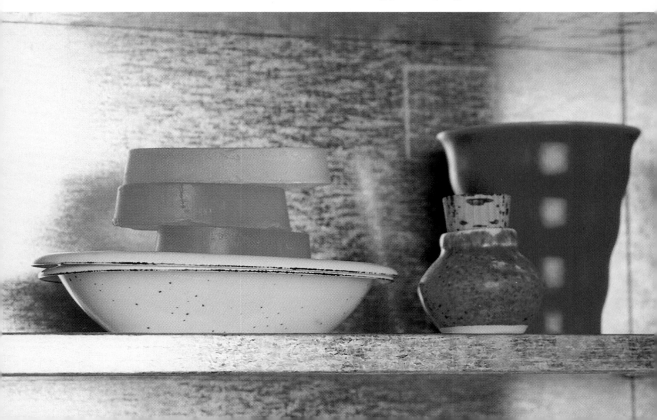

Using the Cutter

Step 1: **Before cutting, fill a spray bottle with water or isopropyl alcohol and lightly moisten the cutter's surface.** This makes for easy, frictionless pushing. The smooth linoleum or Formica top won't mar the surfaces of your soap, and it's easy to clean. You'll also need to secure the cutter so that it doesn't move while you're cutting soap. This can be as easy as having it abut the wall behind your kitchen countertop or clamping it to a table.

When you slide both the top and the bottom blocks, the wire will move back and forth to create any size bar you desire. If the wire doesn't go all the way over to the wooden guide, flip the cutter over. The movable wooden block underneath the cutter probably needs to be rotated. As you push the block of soap through the cutter, try to push it in toward the guide board as well as forward. In other words, concentrate on pushing in a diagonal direction.

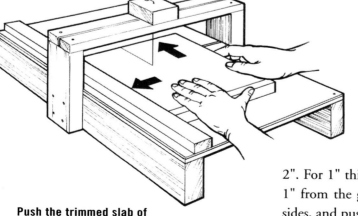

Push the trimmed slab of soap through the wire.

The block of soap can wobble if it's not pushed into the guide, resulting in wavy edges on your soap. Try using a small length of 1" x 2" wood to push the block of soap. It gives you more control, and it eliminates dent marks and fingerprints.

If you constructed the wooden mold described in chapter 3, one recipe will yield a 12" x 12" x 2" slab of soap. Before cutting bars, "clean" the slab. Set the wire about ⅛" from the guide, and gently push the block through. Trim all four sides. Then gently scrape off the flaws on the top and bottom of the block. These trim scraps can be remelted or used as is.

Step 2: **Now the block is ready to be cut into bars.** If you want a 2" x 3" x 1" bar of soap, first take a ruler and measure 2" over from the wooden guide. Jiggle the wire over to this spot, and tighten it if it's slack. Make sure the wire is straight up and down, not at an angle.

Step 3: **Push the trimmed slab through until you're left with six strips 2" wide.**

Step 4: **Now measure 3" from the guide, and move the wire here.** Run the strips through sideways, and cut into 3" lengths. You now have blocks of soap measuring 2" x 3" x 2". For 1" thick bars of soap, set the wire 1" from the guide, flip the bars on their sides, and push them through again.

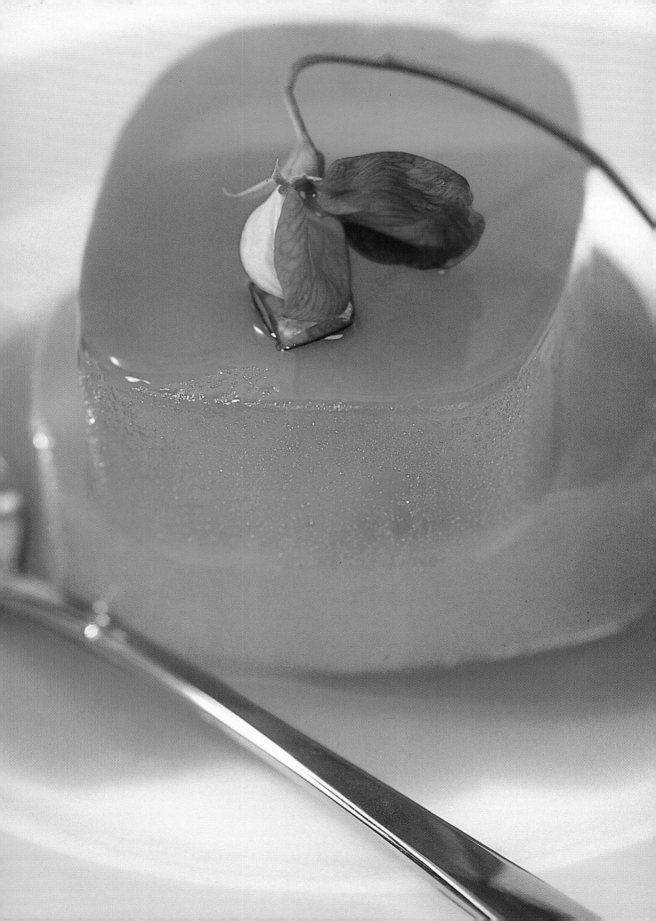

variable-speed drill mixer

This mixer may look a bit primitive, but it works like a dream. If you own a variable-speed drill, it costs next to nothing to make. There will be no plastic tenting to bother with and no manual stirring.

Like the adjustable-wire bar cutter, this mixer is easy to assemble from an assortment of common materials. With this mixer, the only thing necessary to adjust is the stove heat. If you find the tin can setup too primitive, you can purchase drill guides at hardware stores, although they are quite expensive.

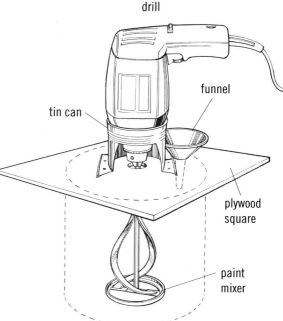

drill

funnel

tin can

plywood square

paint mixer

WHAT YOU'LL NEED

MATERIALS

- 1 square of plywood, sized to cover the entire top of your soap pot. Add an extra inch or two for a little overhang
- 1 tin can, 3" in diameter, 4" high (dog or cat food can size)
- 24 ½" wood screws
- 1 15-gallon paint mixer for ⅜" electric drills, found in hardware or paint supply stores
- 1 variable-speed ⅜" drill with set button
- 1 small funnel

TOOLS

Hand or circular saw
Drill
Tin snips
Pliers
Hacksaw

◄ **These smooth bars of soap are the result of careful scraping and cutting.**

Assembling the Mixer

Step 1: **Cut the plywood to fit over the top of your mixing pot.** Add an inch or two to compensate for any movement of the board during mixing. If your pot is 12" in diameter, cut the plywood in a 14" x 14" square. If you have a jigsaw, cut a circle 14" in diameter.

Step 2: **Measure the center point of the board, and drill a ½" hole.** This hole is for the shaft of the paint stirrer. Then, 4" or 5" out from the center hole, drill a ¾" hole. The neck of a small funnel will fit in here. Drill a third hole ¼" in diameter 3" or 4" out from the center in any direction. This is for the shaft of the thermometer.

Step 3: **Remove the top and bottom of the tin can.** With tin snips, make four ½" cuts equidistant from each other up the side of the can (at 12, 3, 6, and 9 o'clock). Select any two adjacent cuts and continue snipping to within an inch from the top. Snip off the flap formed by these two long cuts. With pliers, bend all the sharp edges in. This will keep fingers from being cut.

Use pliers to gently fold out the remaining three ½" flaps of metal. Tap two holes into each of the three flaps with a hammer and nail.

Step 4: **Set the tin can over the ½" center hole in the plywood.** The middle of the can should sit dead center over the hole. Attach the can to the board by sinking ½" screws into the wood through the holes in the flaps.

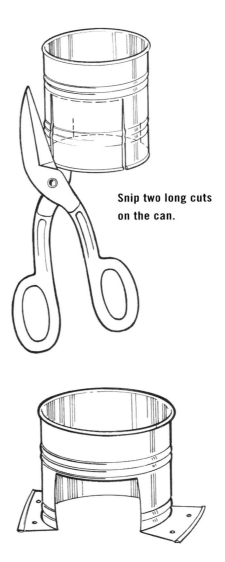

Snip two long cuts on the can.

Fold out the flaps and create screw holes.

Step 5: With the hacksaw, cut the mixing blade to size.

The paint mixers come with 17" shafts — much too long for any mixing pot. Saw so that the blade clears the bottom of the pot by at least ½". Here is an easy way to do this:

➲ First, measure the height of the pot.

➲ To this number add another inch and a half. This will be the approximate length you'll need to cut the mixer blade, as measured from the tip of the stirring end. For instance, if the pot is 7" high, you'll need to saw the mixing blade to 8½". You may need to adjust the blade length with another small cut to get it to fit just right.

PAINT MIXER PRECAUTION

Paint mixers usually come coated with a colored varnish. You might want to take some paint remover and strip this away before you make soap; otherwise, the lye from your soap will dissolve the varnish over time. This varnish is somewhat toxic, but since it takes many mixings to completely dissolve the coating, it probably isn't cause for much concern. The varnish will also faintly tint your finished soap.

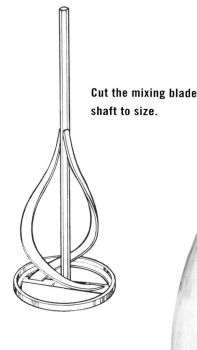

Cut the mixing blade shaft to size.

▶ **Good tools are essential to the creation of every type of soap, from the most basic to the most eye catching.**

Using the Mixer

Step 1: Stick the mixer shaft up through the center hole of the plywood, then lower the tip of the drill into the can.

The cutaway hole on the side of the can enables you to stick the chuck key through and tighten the chuck around the mixing shaft.

Step 2: Before lowering the drill into the liquid, adjust its speed.

For the blending of the oil and lye, run the mixer on medium speed or higher, but not so high that the soap splashes to the top of the pot. For stirring the alcohol and soap, turn the speed to medium low; this prevents the formation of foam, which can be difficult to subdue.

Step 3: The funnel allows you to add ingredients such as lye and sugar solutions with minimal fuss.

Take care to stuff a small wad of plastic wrap into the funnel neck after the addition of the alcohol to help contain the vapors.

The mixer is useful for every stage of transparent soap production, with one exception. You must hand-stir the alcohol into the soap and manually scrape the soap off the sides and bottom of the pot. After the pot's surfaces have been cleaned, turn the mixer back on and proceed.

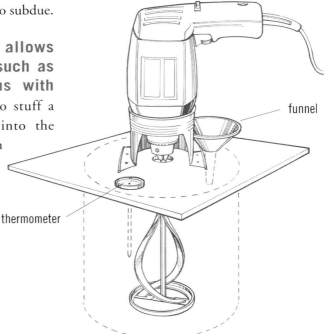

funnel

thermometer

Step 4: **The thermometer rests permanently in its slot so that the temperature can be constantly monitored.** There's no need to manually dip the probe every few minutes, as with hand mixing. If the shaft of the thermometer isn't totally immersed in the liquid, the temperature reading on the dial may register a slightly lower than actual temperature.

To correct for temperature discrepancies, first dip (by hand) the thermometer shaft into the soap stock. Let's say it reads 160°F (70°C). Next, slip the thermometer into its slot on the mixer frame. Set the mixer over the soap pot, and take this temperature. Say it reads 150°F (65°C). You now know that there's a discrepancy of 10°F (12°C), so in the future you'll heat the stock accordingly, without having to hand-dip for an accurate temperature.

Note: The gap between the center hole and the mixer shaft will allow the evaporation of a small amount of alcohol. It shouldn't be cause for much concern, but if you want to seal the gap, create a gasket with a piece of rubber. Cut a small hole in the middle of a 3" x 3" square of thin rubber (an old inner tube or bicycle tube will do), and staple the rubber to the underside of the plywood, aligning the hole in the rubber with the center hole of the plywood.

▼ **In the company of greenery and objects from the sea, this soap completes an artful display.**

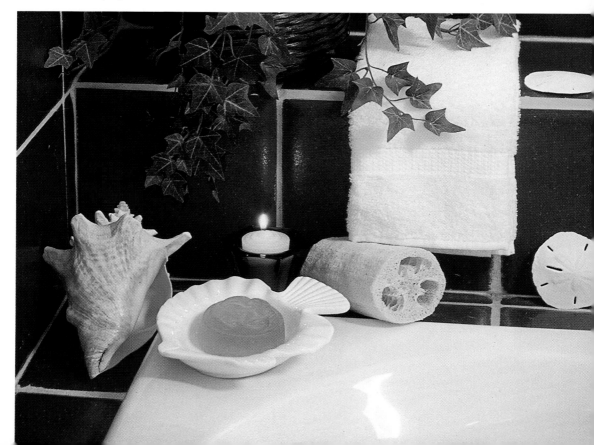

trouble-
⑧ shooting

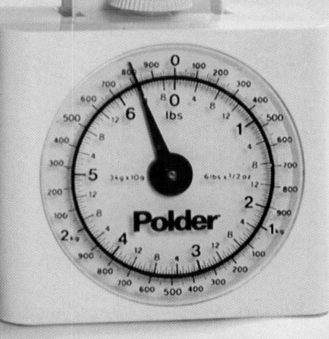

Failure in making soap — either opaque or transparent — is almost always a result of either improper measurement of the ingredients or temperature, or undermixing of the broth. Take care that your scales and thermometers are accurate, and that will eliminate nearly all of the possible problems. One of the beauties of transparent soapmaking is that some problems can be rectified when the soap is in the alcohol solution phase, but that's no license to abandon care and precision. Sometimes no amount of tinkering can right the wrong, and you're stuck with a cloudy batch of soap.

The following list delineates most of the problems you'll encounter, and it offers some possible solutions.

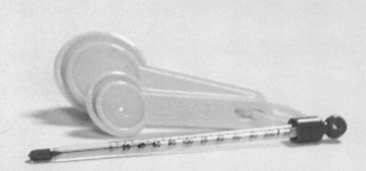

problems & solutions

Problem: Soap mixture doesn't thicken and trace.

Solution: None of the recipes in this book should take much over an hour to trace with manual stirring, so if you're still stirring after 2 hours, read on. Most likely the problem is either too little lye or too much water.

Though there is no way at this point to be absolutely certain of which problem you have, chances are it's the lye, because unless water was added in substantial excess, soap is generally forgiving of a little extra. Try adding a bit more lye solution. Start with 1 ounce of dry caustic soda and mix with 2 ounces of water. Cool it down for a minute or so, then add it to the soap stock.

Mix for another 10 to 15 minutes, and look for signs of tracing. If nothing has happened, add 3 ounces more of lye solution. Stir some more. Unless your initial measurement of caustic soda was terribly off, the soap should trace after two or three of these smaller additions.

A soap stock that's too cool will take a longer time to trace. If your thermometer is accurate, check this possibility off.

The faster the lye and the oil are brought into contact, the quicker they saponify and trace. This is one advantage of electrical mixing over manual. If you don't have a blender, stick blender, or a food processor, borrow one now, and mix.

If none of the above techniques works for your stubborn soap, it's wisest to start again. You might want to pour the discarded mix into a plastic-lined mold and cover it for 24 hours just to see what happens. It could end up hardening into respectable opaque soap.

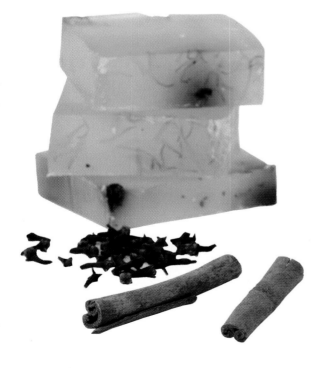

◄ **For visual interest, mix in some herb or spice fragments before you pour the soap into molds.**

Problem: Soap mixture curdles and separates.

Solution: This problem is usually caused by mismeasurement of ingredients or wide variations between the temperatures of the lye and oils. Slow, uneven stirring can also contribute, so try mixing curdled soap with a blender, stick blender, or food processor.

If the batch still remains curdled after blending, it's best to toss it out, because the problem is probably an excess of lye. To correct, see Too Much Lye, Too Little Lye on page 114.

Rosin and stearic acid in an oil mix will curdle even if everything is measured correctly, so don't panic. Just follow directions for their use in chapter 5.

> **Undermixing is another culprit, particularly if you stir by hand.**

▶ **If you plan to use a blender for soapmaking, be sure to purchase a separate machine rather than using your food blender.**

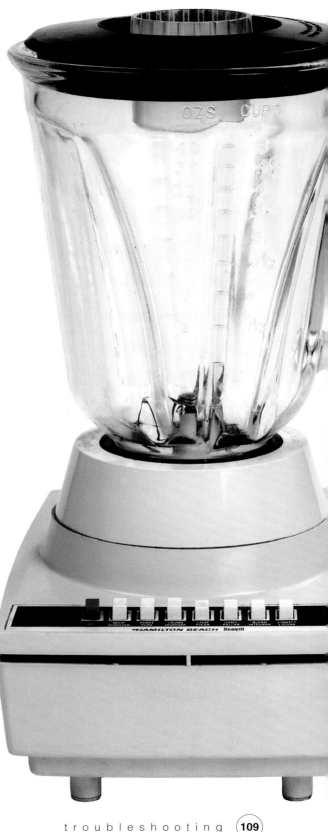

Problem: Soap doesn't gel.

Solution: If your soap traces (you've measured all the ingredients properly) and its temperature is around 135 to 145°F (57–62°C) before you cover the pot, there should be no problem with gelling.

Failure to reach the colloidal state will be due to insufficient or excessive lye, too much water in the stock, or a low temperature.

An excess of lye is usually noticeable in the appearance of the soap after it's rested under the blankets for a while. Good soap will turn hard and pasty before gelling, but if the soap stays pasty and doesn't pass into the gel state, or gels only slightly before firming up again, there's too much lye. Before correcting by using the instructions on page 114, you'll need to dissolve the soap in 2 pounds of ethanol; it will be difficult to stir melted stearic acid into

▼ **You will sometimes encounter problems during the soapmaking process. This doesn't necessarily mean that a batch is ruined.**

hardened soap. Add 2 to 3 ounces of melted stearic acid, then cover the pot with plastic (as per the alcohol/lye method) and place it in a double boiler. Cook the soap at a gentle boil for 15 to 20 minutes.

Without phenolphthalein it can be hard to tell if the soap is still overalkalized, but excess hydroxide will usually cause "splintering" of the cooled soap when it is pressed with a finger. If splintering occurs, add 2 ounces more stearic acid, cover the pot, and return to heat. Continue cooking and adding stearic acid until the cooled soap softens when pressed with a finger. Proceed to adding the glycerin and sugar solution.

A deficiency of lye can possibly be corrected if you follow the instructions given on page 108 for soap that doesn't thicken or trace, providing your soap at this point isn't too thick to stir.

A too-low temperature is the easiest problem to correct. Place the pot over a double boiler, and heat. Use the double-boiler method described in chapter 4.

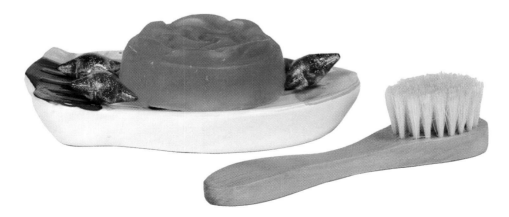

Problem: Soap doesn't dissolve in alcohol.

Solution: The temperature of the alcohol/soap stock needs to be in the range of 150 to 160°F (65–70°C) to dissolve the soap completely. Make sure your thermometer is registering correctly. If the soap has difficulty dissolving after you've stirred it for several minutes at the proper temperature, or if the stock is somewhat thick and viscous, you haven't measured the alcohol correctly.

To correct, add 2 ounces of alcohol at a time, and stir. Keep adding in small increments until all the soap dissolves or any syrupy thickness to the broth is thinned to the viscosity of water.

> Note: Soap stirred in a blend of ethanol and isopropyl alcohol will take longer to dissolve.

Problem: Cloudy soap.

Solution: After you've added the sugar solution, then poured a small test sample only to find that the sample clouds upon hardening, don't worry too much. This cloudiness can almost always be fixed unless your initial measurements of lye and oils were way off.

Usually 4 or 5 extra ounces of solvent will dissipate the cloudiness. If 4 or 5 extra ounces of sugar solution, alcohol, or glycerin don't solve the problem, you'll have to tinker a bit more. Just remember to keep the heat near 160°F (70°C), and be sure to do all your adjustments while the soap is still in the pot, using small tests on glass as your indicators. The transparency of these samples will be identical to that of the finished bars of soap. If there's some cloudiness in the test samples, it won't work to cross your fingers and pour the soap into molds, hoping for the best. Before taking corrective measures, please continue reading this section.

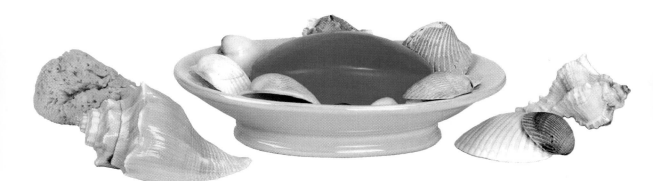

Cloudiness can be caused by any of several conditions:

▶ Not Enough Solvent.

An insufficient amount of alcohol, glycerin, and/or sugar solution is the most likely reason for cloudiness, if your measurements of lye, oils, and temperature were correct. Transparent soap needs a certain amount of these solvents for clarity.

This problem is the easiest to fix. Use sugar solution first, because it produces the best clarity. And it's cheapest.

If your first test sample on glass turns milky, add 3 ounces of sugar solution to the liquid stock, and stir for a half minute to incorporate. Pour another small sample onto glass. If it's still milky, add another 3 ounces and stir again. Don't repeat this procedure more than two times, because excess sugar in the soap can cause softness, sweating, or even cloudiness in the hardened bars. Instead, try adding a few ounces of alcohol. Soap that's still milky after 8 to 10 additional ounces of solvents probably suffers from some other problem, such as mismeasurement of ingredients. If you want to continue adding solvents, be forewarned — too much solvent will prevent the firming up of the soap after it's poured into molds, or will produce soft, sticky bars.

▶ An Excess of Solvents.

Cloudiness can be caused by an excess of solvents as well as by a deficiency of solvents. Perfectly transparent soap seems to exist in a somewhat narrow window, balanced between too little and too much solvent.

A deficiency of solvents usually gives the soap a uniformly hazy appearance. An excess often manifests as soft, sticky soap or soap that doesn't firm up very well. Mottled, blotchy areas surrounded by areas of clear, firm transparent soap are another sign of excess solvents. These blotches are milky and soft and are often more pronounced near the center of a large slab, the reason being that the soap has taken longer to cool there. Slower cooling times promote cloudiness, and excess solvents delay the cooling and hardening of the soap even further.

Overaddition of either glycerin or sugar solution is the likely cause. As mentioned in chapter 2 on ingredients, both of these solvents can cause stickiness or cloudiness when used in excess. An excess of alcohol will not produce this problem. Rosin-based soaps are particularly sensitive to excess sugar. Even 2 or 3 extra ounces of sugar in one of these formulations can cause cloudy areas that grow almost like a bread mold. What begins as a few random white patches goes on to spread and engulf a large slab of soap within three or four days, turning the slab into white pasty mush.

If you think your soft or mottled soap is caused by an excess of solvents, try remelting the soap. Then pour it into smaller molds and flash-cool it in the freezer or refrigerator to render it transparent. This doesn't always work. The best antidote for mushy soap is to first remelt it, then add melted stearic acid and lye solution. In essence, you're adding more soap to the soap. Stearic acid works much more effectively than extra palm oil or coconut oil. It not only produces a harder soap that consequently cools more quickly (thus retard-

ing the formation of crystals) but also saponifies much more rapidly than an oil, requiring less mixing time.

Unfortunately, you can't dribble a test sample on glass and get an accurate reading as to the transparency of the whole batch. This seems to be the one exception to that principle. A small sample cools quickly enough to prevent the formation of the soft spots that will manifest in a larger, more slowly cooling mold. So pour and wait. If you have to remelt the soap a second time, add 3 or 4 ounces of alcohol along with the additional stearic acid and lye solution to compensate for any evaporation.

ADDING EXTRA STEARIC ACID AND LYE

For every ounce of stearic acid added to the remelted soap, add ½ ounce of standard lye solution. The amount of extra stearic acid and lye solution necessary will depend on how blotchy the soap is. There aren't any hard-and-fast rules. If the slab appears only slightly blotched, you might start with 3 or 4 ounces of melted stearic acid. For badly mottled soap, try 7 or 8 ounces. Add it to the 160°F (70°C) soap stock, stir for 10 to 15 minutes, settle, then repour into the molds.

▶ Too Much Lye, Too Little Lye.

This is where phenolphthalein really comes in handy. When dropped onto a sample of soap, it allows you to assess the situation immediately. For instructions, see Using Phenolphthalein on page 42.

Old-time soapmakers didn't have phenolphthalein and relied instead on squeezing the hardened sample with their fingers. Here is their simple method: Press your finger into the milky sample. If it splinters into numerous small sharp-edged pieces, the lye is in excess. A milky sample that feels soft and greasy and flattens out under pressure is a sign of too little lye.

If the test indicates an excess of lye, proceed with this technique: Melt a few ounces of stearic acid. Add 1 to 2 ounces to the stock, cover pot, and return to the double boiler for 15 to 20 minutes. Keep the temperature steady at 160°F (70°C). Saponification is resuming, and time is needed for neutralization of the stearic acid and lye. After 20 minutes, scoop out a sample and test again. If the sample is still milky, repeat the process. Continue adding stearic acid until the mixture tests clear.

If the soap-squeezing test indicates too little lye, mix up some extra lye solution. This doesn't have to be accurately weighed. Pour ¼ cup of dry caustic soda into ½ cup of distilled water, and stir. Add 1 to 2 ounces of this solution to the soap stock, cover with plastic, and then place in the double boiler. Stir or boil gently for 20 minutes, and then test again. If the sample remains soft and greasy, add 1 to 2 ounces more of the lye solution and cook for another 15 to 20 minutes. Continue this process until the cooled sample tests clear and feels firm under pressure from your fingertips.

▶ Incomplete saponification.

There's a good chance cloudiness will result if you don't allow the soap enough time in the gel state. This is a crucial phase, when the fatty acids and lye are reacting and neutralizing. If your soap takes longer than an hour to gel, wait until it does. Then stir, and cover it for an hour. Another option is to use the double-boiler method outlined on page 40. If it hasn't gelled after 3 hours something is wrong — probably your measurements of oil and/or lye.

A FINAL WORD ON CLOUDINESS

Cloudiness can sometimes appear in the liquid soap stock even after the soap has completely dissolved in alcohol. Test the pH — the cloudiness is probably due to an excess or deficiency of lye or undercooking of the soap. Correct for this by using the procedure outlined on this page. Contaminated ingredients can also cause this problem.

▶ **Over-Evaporation of the Alcohol.** If you let the temperature of the alcohol and soap stock rise much above 160 or 170°F (70–76°C) for extended periods of time, or if your pot isn't well covered, the alcohol will evaporate quickly. Some evaporation during mixing is inevitable, but beyond a certain point, enough is lost to cause cloudiness in the finished bar. It's a difficult problem to diagnose. One trick that works (providing that you are absolutely certain you measured everything correctly) is to add up all the weights in the written recipe, then weigh your cloudy stock. Compare the two numbers. If the weight of the stock is substantially lower than the weight of the recipe, add more alcohol.

Note: You won't have to make up the entire difference with alcohol. A portion of the difference will be enough to restore clarity, so add incrementally, 2 to 3 ounces at a time. Stir for a minute or so after each addition, enough to ensure thorough incorporation into the stock. Sample on glass each time.

▶ **Contamination.** Several substances can contaminate your soap and cause it to turn cloudy:

Undissolved soap. Make sure that the soap and alcohol stock is heated to 160°F (70°C) and stirred long enough to dissolve the soap. Undissolved soap appears as odd-sized opaque bits surrounded by clearer soap. Try remelting and stirring for another 15 minutes.

Problem: White spots that "grow."

Solution: Within a day or two after pouring your soap, do you notice small white spots that appear feathery around the edges? Do these spots grow over the course of the next few days, eventually forming large white areas of mushy, opaque soap?

This problem is due to insoluble fatty acid soaps, specifically soaps formed from stearic and palmitic acids. Stearic- and palmitic-based oils, such as palm and tallow, form the hardest soaps, and are consequently the least soluble. If these soaps aren't completely dissolved by alcohol, they can trigger a crystalline "chain reaction." This is what's happening when the white spots grow like a mold or fungus, engulfing much or all of the transparent soap mass.

Why do some batches of transparent soap crystallize and others don't? It may be caused by soap that wasn't allowed enough time to dissolve in the alcohol bath. Or it may be due to palm oil or tallow that contains excessively high levels of stearic and palmitic acid.

When molten palm oil and tallow are pumped into large containers, the oil cools into layers or "fractions." Lighter, more soluble fatty acids float to the top and heavier, more insoluble fatty acids sink. Because of this, the bottom of a 55-gallon drum of oil may contain enough extra stearic or palmitic acid to supersaturate a transparent soap stock. If you buy palm oil or tallow in 5-gallon pails, melt the oil and stir before using. This will help avoid the wider variations in oil fractions. Check with your supplier, too — make certain that they agitate the melted oils in their drums or tanks before pumping it into smaller containers.

To correct the "flowering" caused by insoluble soaps, remelt the soap and cook for another 20 to 30 minutes, using a plastic sheeting "cap" as described in the Alcohol/Lye Method in chapter 4. Add 3 to 4 additional ounces of alcohol, as well. If the soap cools and forms white spots again, remelt and add an additional 4 to 6 ounces of a 1:1 alcohol–lye solution. The flowering will probably disappear with increased levels of solvent, but your finished soap will be slightly softer and dissolve more quickly.

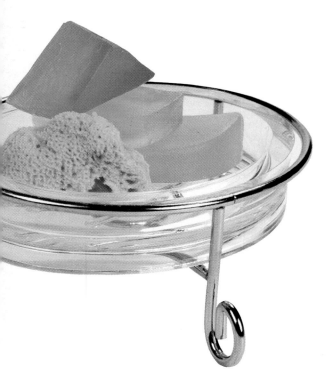

Problem: Soap doesn't harden in molds.

Solution: Your soap should take no longer than 12 hours to firm up, but if it hasn't done so within this time, give it another day or so.

None of the recipes in this book will have difficulty setting. If any do, perhaps you've over-added solvents while trying to correct for cloudiness, or maybe you've mismeasured ingredients. If the soap hasn't firmed up after 24 hours in the mold, you could try remelting it, then adding a few ounces of melted stearic acid and lye to act as a hardener. See the section on an excess of solvents (page 113) for the procedure on adding extra stearic acid and lye.

Problem: Sticky, cloudy top layer.

Solution: If your hardened bars have a sticky, cloudy layer on top and a clear, firm, transparent layer beneath, your soap has either an excess of oil or a deficiency of lye.

You can try remelting this kind of soap and adding a bit more lye solution. Follow the instructions given in the section on tracing (page 108). If the layer isn't too thick, the addition of extra lye will probably eliminate it.

Don't expect as much success if the layers are thicker and more pronounced. If corrective measures don't solve the problem, skim off the sticky layer — it can always be used to wash dishes.

◄ **With a bit of adjustment, even a problematic soap batch will turn out gorgeous.**

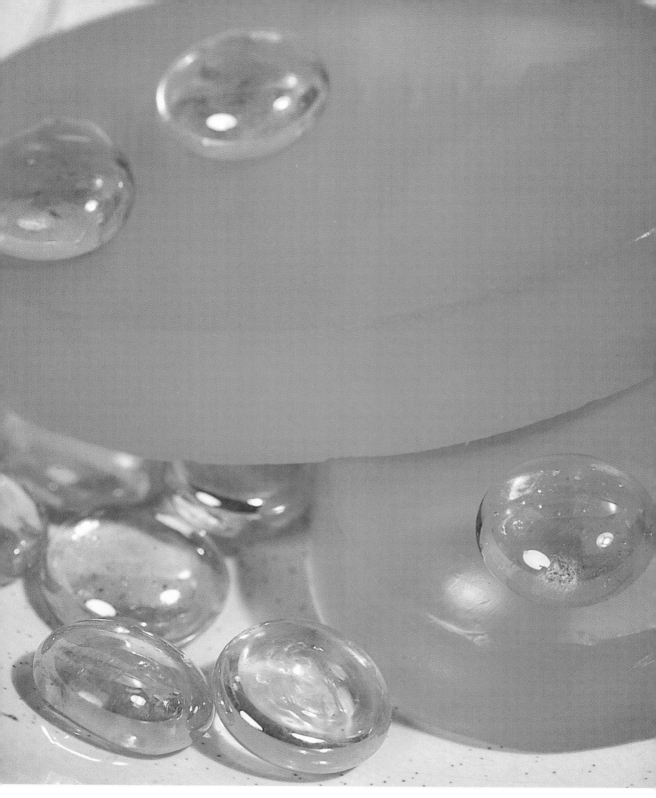

▲ Become familiar with the various potential problems before you begin making soap; this will help you make informed decisions when the need for corrections arises.

Bibliography

Davidsohn, J., E. J. Better, and A. Davidsohn. *Soap Manufacture,* Volume 1. New York: Interscience Publishers, Inc., 1953.

Gathmann, Henry. *American Soaps.* Chicago: Henry Gathmann, 1893.

Kuntom, Ainie, et al., "Transparent/ Translucent Soap Derived From Palm Oil." Paper read at the ABISA Congress, October 1992, Olinda, Brazil.

Osteroth, David. "Transparent Soaps." *Dragoco Report,* November/December, 1979.

Thomssen, E. G., and Kemp, C. R. *Modern Soap Making.* New York: MacNair-Dorland Co., 1937.

Whalley, George. "See-Through Soaps." *Household and Personal Products Industry,* July, 1993.

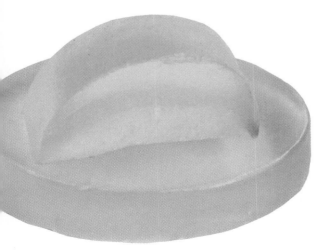

Glossary

Alkali. Any hydroxide or carbonate with basic properties, soluble in water and able to neutralize acids. In soapmaking, sodium or potassium hydroxide neutralizes fatty acids.

Cold-process. A soapmaking technique that relies almost exclusively on the heat generated by the chemical reaction of fatty acids and alkali to produce soap. No external heat is applied once the ingredients have been mixed.

Colloid. A gel-like substance made up of very small, insoluble particles larger than molecules but small enough so that they remain suspended in a fluid medium. All soap exists in a colloidal state during part of saponification. Transparent soap is soap held in this colloidal state through the addition of certain solvents such as alcohol and glycerin.

Distilled water. Water that results from boiling, then condensation of the steam, to remove any mineral or other impurities.

Efflorescence. A term used in transparent soapmaking to describe a milkiness or gradual clouding of the soap's transparency.

Essential oil. A volatile oil steamed or pressed from the fruits, flowers, stems, or roots of plants; used especially for perfumes, soaps, and flavorings.

Ethanol, or ethyl alcohol. The primary alcohol used in the production of transparent soap, produced from the fermentation of carbohydrates. It is clear, colorless, and very flammable.

Fatty acids. Along with glycerides, fatty acids are the main constituents of animal and vegetable fats. Fatty acids react chemically with the alkalis to form soap. There are many kinds of fatty acids, and each has distinct properties, which in turn affect the characteristics of the soap produced from them.

Fragrance oil. A laboratory-produced synthetic version of a true essential oil or a natural fragrance, such as peach. Fragrance oils are often a combination of both synthetic and true essential oils.

Full-boiled. A soapmaking process in which the oils and caustic solution are combined, then heated in steam kettles to the boiling point. This allows for the most complete neutralization of free fatty acids and alkalis, and is the process used by large-scale soap manufacturers.

Glycerin. A thick, sweet-tasting, clear fluid that is actually an alcohol. A by-product of soap manufacture, it can also be produced synthetically from propylene, a petroleum by-product. Used as an emollient, a humectant, and a primary solvent in the manufacture of transparent soaps.

Hard fat. Any animal or vegetable fat that is solid at room temperature; largely composed of the fatty acids stearin and palmitin. Palm oil and tallow are the two most common hard fats used for soapmaking.

Humectant. A substance used to preserve moisture content. The humectant glycerin combined with rose water is the earliest known lotion.

Isopropyl alcohol. A petroleum-derived alcohol sometimes used as a partial substitute for ethyl alcohol in transparent soapmaking.

pH. Standing for the "potential of hydrogen," a term used to indicate acidity or alkalinity. A pH of 7, or the value of pure water, is regarded as neutral. Acids have a pH below 7; alkalis, above 7. "Neutral" soap, however, has a pH of approximately 9.5, or alkaline.

Phenolphthalein. A chemical compound used as an acid-base indicator, turning pink in the presence of an alkali and remaining colorless in a solution containing acid.

Potassium hydroxide. Also known as caustic potash. A strong alkali; when combined with a fatty acid it produces liquid soap.

Rendering. The process by which tallow (beef fat) is boiled in water to remove the impurities. The cleaned fat is then used for soapmaking.

Rosin. The pale yellow residue remaining after the volatile oils are distilled from the oleoresin of pine trees. Rosin acts as a preservative and greatly enhances the transparency of the soap.

Saponification. The chemical reaction that converts a fatty acid and an alkali into soap and glycerin.

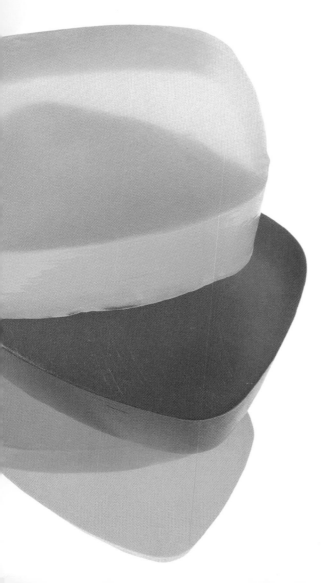

Semi-boiled. One of three basic soap-making processes. Oils and a caustic solution are mixed, then heated to between 140° and 160°F (59–70°C). Transparent soap is made using the semi-boiled method.

Soap. Along with glycerin, soap is the by-product of a chemical reaction involving fatty acids and caustic soda or potash. Soap is actually a salt.

Sodium hydroxide. Also known as caustic soda, one of two primary alkalis used in the production of soap. Combined with a fatty acid it produces a hard soap.

Soft oil. An oil that is liquid at room temperature, usually characterized by a high percentage of the unsaturated fatty acids oleic acid and linoleic acid. Olive, canola, and cottonseed oil are soft oils. Castor oil is the soft oil of choice for transparent soapmaking because of its ability to act as a solvent. It is characterized by a high percentage of ricinoleic acid.

Solvent. A liquid capable of dissolving or dispersing another substance. Alcohol, glycerin, water, and sugar solutions are all solvents used to hold soap in a colloidal state for the purpose of rendering opaque soap transparent.

Transparency. Soap is officially termed transparent if 14-point typeface can be read clearly through a ¼-inch-thick slice of soap.

Resources

Angel's Earth Natural Product Ingredients
1633 Scheffer Avenue
St. Paul, MN 55116-1427
(651) 698-3601
Fax: (651) 698-3636
E-mail: a-earth@pconline.com
Vegetable oils, sulfonated castor oil, jojoba, preservatives, essential and fragrance oils, dyes, lanolin, glycerin, citric acid, rosin, containers.

Aroma Creations, Inc.
24691 State Route 20
Sedro Woolley, WA 98284-8015
(360) 854-9000
Fax: (360) 856-4384
E-mail: aroma@gte.net
Fragrance oils, essential oils.

Aromystique, Inc.
P.O. Box 248
Granbury, TX 76048
(888) 722-1244
Fax: (817) 573-2545
Web site: www.aromystique.com
E-mail: dgutmann@aromystique.com
Vegetable oils, essential and fragrance oils, containers.

**Blue Moon Botanicals Natural Soap
and Body Care**
33144 Five Points Road
Kingston, IL 60145
(815) 784-5861
E-mail: B1MoonB@aol.com
Contact person: Helen Dubovik
Blue Moon Botanicals, founded in 1996, provides all-natural aromatherapy soaps and body care. Self-indulgence for body and spirit.

Brambleberry
Bay Street Village
301 W. Holly, space 11&12
Bellingham, WA 98225
(360) 738-8382
Fax: (360) 738-5810
Web site: www.brambleberry.com
E-mail: bramblebery@prodigy.net
Vegetable oils, preservatives, essential and fragrance oils, containers, glycerin, citric acid, soap molds, melt-and-pour supplies.

Camden-Grey Essential Oils
7178A S.W. 47th Street
Miami, FL 33155
(305) 740-3494
Fax: (305) 740-8242
Web site: www.camdengrey.com
E-mail: aroma@bellsouth.net
Vegetable oils, essential oils, glycerin, citric acid, preservatives, containers.

Cat's Paw Enterprises
2333 Cape George Road
Port Townsend, WA 98368
(360) 385-3407
Contact person: Diana Johnson
Diana makes and sells goat milk soaps and water-based soaps, and creates custom soapmaking kits. Her products cater to people with sensitive skin types and those with allergies.

Chem Lab Supplies
1060-C Ortega Way
Placentia, CA 92870
(714) 630-7902
Fax: (714) 630-3553
Web site: www.chemlab.com
E-mail: info@chemlab.com
Vegetable oils, sulfonated castor oil, lanolin, essential and fragrance oils, preservatives, dyes, glycerin, citric acid, sodium and potassium hydroxide, containers, phenolphthalein, rosin.

Country Scentuals
21201 Pecan Valley Road
Newalla, OK 74857
(405) 386-6914
Web site: www.countryscentuals.com
E-mail: Reneerenee@aol.com
Contact person: Renee Thompson
Country Scentuals is an all-natural soap and toiletries company dedicated to creating the most luxurious bath products without the use of harsh chemicals.

Cranberry Lane Natural Beauty Products
65-2710 Barnet Highway
Coquitlam, B.C. Canada V3B1B8
(604) 944-1488
Fax: (604) 944-1439
Web site: www.cranberrylane.com
E-mail: staff@cranberrylane.com
Vegetable oils, rosin, sulfonated castor oil, essential oils, dyes, preservatives, glycerin, citric acid, phenolphthalein, containers, soap molds.

Delaware City Soap Company
P.O. Box 4112
Delaware City, DE 19706
(302) 832-2696
Web site: www.delcitysoap.com
E-mail: info@delcitysoap.com
Contact person: Rebecca Keilor
Located in a beautiful and historic riverfront town, this company specializes in authentic recreations of classic nineteenth-century soaps using fine vegetable ingredients and essential oils.

Designs By AnnaLiese
1430 N.W. 11th Street
Corvallis, OR 97330
Phone/fax: (541) 753-7881
E-mail: Designs ByA@aol.com
Contact person: AnnaLiese M. Moran

The Essential Oil Company
1719 S.E. Umatilla Street
Portland, OR 97202
(800) 729-5912
Fax: (503) 872-8767
Web site: http://essentialoil.com
Vegetable oils, lanolin, essential and fragrance oils, preservatives, glycerin, containers, soap molds.

Flower Moon Soaps
8192 Bakers Lane
Chestertown, MD 21620
(410) 778-2385
Contact persons: Lisa and Matt Redman
Flower Moon Soaps makes soaps of unusual color and textures, using high-quality oils and a unique blending of fragrances for scents.

Frontier Natural Products Co-op
3021 78th Street
Norway, IA 52318
(800) 669-3275
Fax: (315) 227-7966
Web site: www.frontiercoop.com
E-mail: pat.bayles@frontiercoop.com
Vegetable oils, essential and fragrance oils, lanolin, glycerin, dyes, preservatives, containers.

Gentler Thymes Soap Co.
P.O. Box 284
Palos Heights, IL 60463
Web site: www.soapmaker.com/supplies
E-mail: supplies@soapmaker.com
Contact person: Mary Byerly
Gentler Thymes Soap has been selling handmade cold-process soap since 1995.

Georgie's Ceramic & Clay Co.
756 N.E. Lombard
Portland, OR 97211
(503) 283-1353
Web site: www.georgies.com
E-mail: alan@georgies.com
Fragrance oils, glycerin, dyes, containers, soap molds, melt-and-mold supplies. Check their Web site for information on their Beaverton and Eugene stores.

Gingham 'n' Spice, Ltd./My Sweet Victoria
P.O. Box 88cf
Gardenville, PA 18926
(215) 348-3595
Fax: (215) 348-8021
Web site: www.fragrancesupplies.com
E-mail: robinnoelle@aol.com
Contact person: Nancy Booth
Bottles, essential and fragrance oils, glycerin, and other soap supplies.

Herbal Accents
560 N. Coast Highway 101, Suite 4-A
Encinitas, CA 92024
(760) 633-4255
Fax: (760) 632-7279
Web site: www.herbalaccents.com
E-mail: herbal@herbalaccents.com
Vegetable oils, essential and fragrance oils, potassium hydroxide, glycerin, citric acid, preservatives, dyes, containers, melt-and-pour supplies.

Homesong Handcrafted Soaps
5220 Zimmer Road
Williamston, MI 48895
(517) 655-4037
Web site: www.MIcrafts.com
E-mail: Trish4000@ aol.com
Contact person: Trisha Walton

Indiana Botanic Gardens
3401 W. 37th Avenue
Hobart, IN 46342
(888) 315-3077 (wholesale)
(800) 644-8327
Fax: (219) 947-4148
Web site: www.botanichealth.com
E-mail: wholesale@bontanichealth.com
Vegetable oils, fragrance and essential oils.

Indian River Creations
1843 Cadillac Circle South
Melbourne, FL 32935
Web site: www.handcraftedsoap.com
E-mail: graybeal@digital.net
Contact person: Debby Graybeal
Every uniquely scented soap from Indian River
Creations has a purpose, including antibacterial,
disinfecting, relaxing, or energizing.

Iowa Natural Soapworks
11 W. 16th Street
Davenport, IA 52804
Voice/fax/orders: (800) 265-5252
Web site: www.IowaNaturalSoapworks.com
E-mail: jasidney@revealed.net
Contact person: Jill Sidney
Iowa Natural Soapworks soap is a high-quality, hand-
crafted, natural soap that provides the softest, mildest,
most luxurious moisturizing lather that cleans and
mildly scents.

Janca's Jojoba Oil & Seed Co
456 E. Juanita #7
Mesa, AZ 85204
(480) 497-9494
Fax: (480) 497-1312
E-mail: Jancas3@aol.com
Vegetable oils, essential and fragrance oils, potassium
hydroxide, sulfonated castor oil, glycerin, citric acid,
preservatives, containers.

Liberty Natural Products
8120 S.E. Stark Street
Portland, OR 97215
(800) 298-8427
Fax: (503) 256-1182
Web site: www.libertynatural.com
E-mail: sales@libertynatural.com
Vegetable oils, essential oils, sulfonated castor oil,
preservatives, glycerin, citric acid, dyes, containers,
soap molds, melt-and-pour supplies.

The Loom Rat
369 Stonyhill Drive
Chalfont, PA 18914
E-mail: bobnkate@comcat.com
Contact person: Bob McDaniel
The Loom Rat features Dr. Bob's Herbal Soaps, made
from skin-friendly aromatherapy-type oils, bath salts,
and powders, as well as custom hand-woven accessories
from the loom of The Loom Rat.

LorAnn Oils Inc.
4518 Aurelius Road
Lansing, MI 48910
Mailing address:
P.O. Box 22009
Lansing, MI 48909
Web site: www.lorannoils.com
Vegetable oils, sulfonated castor oil, essential and
fragrance oils, rosin, glycerin, citric acid.

Majestic Mountain Sage
880 North 1430 West
Orem, UT 84057
(801) 227-0837
Fax: (801) 785-8632
Web site: www.the-sage.com
E-mail: info@the-sage.com
Vegetable oils, fragrance and essential oils, phenolph-
thalein, glycerin, citric acid, dyes, containers.

Milky Way Molds
PMB #473
4326 S.E. Woodstock
Portland, OR 97206
(800) 588-7930
(503) 774-4157
Fax: (503) 777-6584
Web site: www.milkywaysoapmolds.com
E-mail: sales@milkywaysoapmolds.com
Soap molds.

Mystic Mountain Soap Crafters
5564 Cool Brook
Montreal, Quebec, Canada H3X 2L5
Phone/fax: (514) 731-2869
Web site: www.mysticsoap.com
E-mail: info@mysticsoap.com
Vegetable oils, essential and fragrance oils, sulfonated
castor oil, glycerin, citric acid, dyes, preservatives, rosin,
phenolphthalein, containers.

Natural Impulse Handmade Soap and Sundries
P.O. Box 94441
Birmingham, AL 35220-4441
(877) IMPULSE
Web site: www.naturalimpulse.com
E-mail: karen@naturalimpulse.com
Contact person: Karen White
Luxurious soaps, handcrafted from all-natural veg-
etable oils. Colorful and rich with scent, skin-friendly,
and gentle on the environment, they're a luxury anyone
can afford!

North Country Mercantile

Box 5368
West Lebanon, NH 03784
(603) 795-2843
Web site: www.northcountrymercantile.com
E-mail: northcountry@esosoft.com
*Vegetable oils, essential and fragrance oils, containers,
soap molds.*

Nurnberg Scientific

6310 S.W. Virginia
Portland, OR 97201
(503) 246-8297
Fax: (503) 246-0360
Web site: www.nurnberg.com
E-mail: sales@nurnberg.com
*Vegetable oils, essential and fragrance oils, glycerin,
potassium hydroxide, rosin, preservatives, phenolph-
thalein.*

Penta Manufacturing Co., Inc.

P.O. Box 1448
Fairfield, NJ 07004
(973) 740-2300
Fax: (973) 740-1839
E-mail: www.pentamfg@msn.com
*Vegetable oils, fragrance and essential oils, glycerin,
potassium hydroxide, rosin, glycerin, citric acid, preser-
vatives, dyes, phenolphthalein.*

The Petal Pusher

17623 53rd Drive N.W.
Stanwood, WA 98292
(360) 652-4367
Fax: (360) 654-0145
Web site: www.thepetalpusher.com/supplies.
  html
E-mail: info@thepetalpusher.com
Contact person: Kathy Tarbox
*Handcrafted botanical soap, vegetable oils, essential
and fragrance oils, glycerin, citric acid, dyes, containers.*

Pharmco Products, Inc.

56 Vale Road
Brookfield, CT 06804-3967
(800) 243-5360
Fax: (203) 740-3481
Web site: www.pharmco-prod.com
E-mail: Pharmco-prod@worldnet.att.net
*5-gallon containers of SDA-3A (denatured alcohol),
1 per year without permit.*

Pisces Rising Aromatherapy Arts and Crafts

1631 N. Colorado
Indianapolis, IN 46218
(317) 375-1718
Web site: http://pages.prodigy.net/ewinslow/
  pisces.htm
E-mail: ewinslow@prodigy.net
Contact person: Ethel Winslow
*Pisces Rising Aromatherapy Arts and Crafts was estab-
lished in 1993 to provide all-natural personal care
products and educate the public about aromatherapy.*

Poya Naturals Inc.

50-4 Van Kirk Drive
Brampton, Ontario, Canada L7A 1C7
(877) 255-7692
Fax: (905) 846-1784
Web site: www.poyanaturals.com
E-mail: deccan@interlog.com
Essential oils.

Pretty Baby Herbal Soap Company

P.O. Box 555
China Grove, NC 28023
(800) 673-8167
Soapmaking kits.

Rainbow Meadow Inc.

5234 Southern Boulevard, Suite F3
Boardman, OH 44512
(800) 207-4047
Fax: (800) 219-0213
E-mail: orders@rainboxmeadow.com
*Vegetable oils, essential oils, glycerin, citric acid, preser-
vatives, dyes, containers, phenolphthalein, soap molds,
melt-and-pour supplies.*

Scentsables

23813 N.E. Canyon Loop
Battle Ground, WA 98604
(360) 687-3502
Web site: www.angelfire.com/biz/NaturalSoaps/
  index.html
E-mail: naturalsoaps@angelfire.com
Contact person: Maggie Anderson
*Scentsables creates herbal and vegetable-based soaps
in small batches using the cold-process method. Many
contain fragrant ground herbs, herbal extracts, and
essential oils.*

Serenity Soaps and Herb Gardens

630 West Dodge Road
Camano Island, WA 98292
(360) 387-0727
E-mail: serenity@greatnorthern.net
Contact person: Sharon Dodge

Shay & Co., Inc.
8535 N. Lombard Street, #202
Portland, OR 97203
(503) 289-5503
Fax: (503) 283-6377
Web site: ironman.linkport.com/~wshay1
E-mail: wshayl@linkport.com
Vegetable oils, preservatives, melt-and-pour supplies.

Simple Pleasures
P.O. Box 194
Old Saybrook, CT 06475
Phone/fax: (860) 395-0085
Web site: http://members.aol.com/pigmntlady/
E-mail: PitmntLady@aol.com
Dyes.

Snowdrift Farm Natural Products
P. O. Box 958
Jefferson, ME 04348-0958
(888) 999-6950 or (207) 549-5905
Web site: www.snowdriftfarm.com
E-mail: whatsnew@snowdriftfarm.com
Contact names: Bill and Trina Wallace
Snowdrift Farm, in south central Maine, provides handmade soaps from all-natural products, as well as supplying essential oils and raw materials to soap and toiletry makers. They carry vegetable oils, essential oils, potassium hydroxide, citric acid, dyes, and containers.

SoapBerry Lane
P.O. Box 65551
Virginia Beach, VA 23467
(757) 490-8852
Web site: www.soapberrylane.com
E-mail: soapberyln@aol.com
Dyes, glycerin, fragrance oils, soap molds, melt-and-pour supplies.

The Soap Box
424 Third Street West
Cochrane, Alberta, Canada TOL 0W1
(403) 932-4530
E-mail: customde@cadvision.com
Contact person: Donna Ramsey
The Soap Box sells all the ingredients for soapmaking, fizzy-o-therapy (bath bombs), lotions, creams, lip balms, and many hard-to-find natural bath and body products.

Soap Crafters Company
2944 S.W. Temple
Salt Lake City, UT 84115
(801) 484-5121
Fax: (801) 487-1958
Web site: www.soapcrafters.com
E-mail: pam@soapcrafters.com
Vegetable oils, essential and fragrance oils, soap molds, melt-and-pour supplies.

Wholesale Supplies Plus.com, Inc.
8611 Whippoorwill Lane
Parma, OH 44130
(800) 359-0944
Web site: www.wholesalesuppliesplus.com
E-mail: catalog@aol.com
Essential and fragrance oils, glycerin, dyes, containers, soap molds, melt-and-pour supplies.

Soapscope
157 Glendale Avenue
Toronto, Ontario, Canada M6R 2T4
(888) 340-5877
Fax: (416) 588-8734
Web site: www.soapscope.com
E-mail: soap@soapscope.com
Palm oil, essential and fragrance oils, citric acid, soap molds, melt-and-pour supplies.

The Soap Saloon
5710 Auburn Boulevard #6
Sacramento, CA 95841
(916) 334-4894
Fax: (916) 334-4897
Web site: www.soapsaloon.com
E-mail: carolyn@soapsaloon.com
Vegetable oils, essential and fragrance oils, glycerin, citric acid, preservatives, dyes, soap molds.

Southern Soap Company
3205 Walker Chapel Road
Fultondale, AL 35068
(800) 723-7627
Web site: www.southernsoapcompany.com
E-mail: SouthSoap@aol.com
Contact person: Tammy Hawk

Squeaky Clean . . . Naturally!
P.O. Box 170
Circleville, NY 10919
(914) 692-7276
Web site: www.squeaky-clean.com
E-mail: soapdoc@squeaky-clean.com
Contact person: Darlene Nielsen
*Why not do something nice for your skin today?
Squeaky Clean offers some of the finest quality hand-
crafted goat's milk soap on the market. Mention this
book for a free sample (while supplies last)!*

Stevenson-Cooper, Inc.
1039 W. Venango Street
P.O. Box 46345
Philadelphia, PA 19160
(888) 420-1663
Fax: (215) 223-3597
Vegetable oils, tallow, rosin.

Sugar Plum Sundries
2101 S. Greenwood Avenue Suite E
Chattanooga, TN 37404
Phone/fax: (423) 624-4511
Web site: www.sugarplum.net
E-mail: info@sugarplum.net
*Vegetable oils, essential oils, potassium hydroxide, citric
acid, preservatives.*

Summers Past Farms Ye Olde Soap Shoppe
15602 Olde Highway 80
Flinn Springs, CA 92021
(619) 390-3525
Fax: (619) 390-7148
Web site: www.soapmaking.com
E-mail: farmsup@aol.com
*Vegetable oils, fragrance and essential oils, potassium
hydroxide, glycerin, citric acid, preservatives, dyes, soap
molds, containers.*

SunCoast Soaps & Supplies
12415 Haley Street
Sun Valley, CA 91352
Phone/fax: (818) 252-1452
E-mail: DeptMW@suncoastsoaps.com
*Vegetable oils, fragrance oils, dyes, containers, soap
molds.*

Sunfeather Natural Soap Co.
1551 Highway 72
Potsdam, NY 13676
Phone/fax: (315) 265-3648
Web site: www.sunsoap.com
E-mail: sunsoap@slic.com
*Vegetable oils, essential oils, glycerin, preservatives,
dyes, soap molds.*

Sweet Cakes Soapmaking Supplies
249 North Road
Kinnelon, NJ 07405
(973) 492-7406
Fax: (973) 992-7413
Web site: www.sweetcakes.com
E-mail: suprphat@aol.com
Fragrance oils.

TKB Trading
356 24th Street
Oakland, CA 94612
(510) 451-9011
Fax: (510) 839-9967
Web site: www.tkbtrading.com
E-mail: tkbtrading@aol.com
*Vegetable oils, essential and fragrance oils, glycerin,
rosin, sulfonated castor oil, preservatives, dyes, citric
acid, phenolphthalein, containers, soap molds, melt-
and-pour supplies.*

Tom Thumb Workshops
10 Holly Street
Onancock, VA 23417
(757) 787-9596
Fax: (757) 787-3136
Web site: www.tomthumbworkshops.com
E-mail: tomthumbworkshps@esva.net
*Vegetable oils, essential and fragrance oils, glycerin,
containers.*

Uncommon Scents
P.O. Box 1941
Eugene, OR 97440
(800) 426-4336
Fax: (888) 343-8196
Web site: http://uncommonscents.net
E-mail: sales@uncommonscents.com
*Vegetable oils, essential and fragrance oils, preserva-
tives, containers.*

Zenith Supplies
6300 Roosevelt Way N.E.
Seattle, WA 98115
(206) 525-7997
Fax: (206) 525-3703
Web site: www.zenithsupplies.com
*Vegetable oils, essential and fragrance oils, glycerin,
citric acid, dyes, containers, soap molds, melt-and-pour
supplies.*

Index

Page numbers in **boldface** indicate charts.

CONVERTING RECIPE MEASUREMENTS TO METRIC

Use the following chart for converting U.S. measurements to metric. Since the conversions are not exact, it's important to convert the measurements for all of the ingredients to maintain the same proportions as the original recipe.

To convert to	When the measurement given is	Multiply it by
milliliters	teaspoons	4.93
milliliters	tablespoons	14.79
milliliters	fluid ounces	29.57
milliliters	cups	236.59
liters	cups	0.236
milliliters	pints	473.18
liters	pints	0.473
milliliters	quarts	946.36
liters	quarts	0.946
liters	gallons	3.785
grams	ounces	28.35
kilograms	pounds	0.454
centimeters	inches	2.54
degrees Celsius	degrees Fahrenheit	⅝ (°−32)

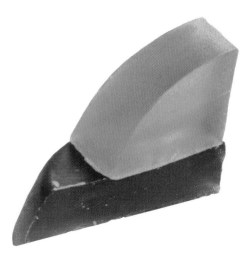

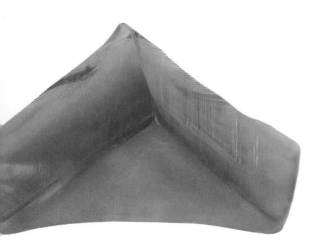

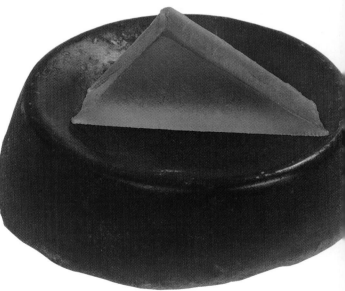

Other Storey Books You Will Enjoy

Making Natural Liquid Soaps, by Catherine Failor. This comprehensive book includes step-by-step instructions for the crafting process, coloring, and scenting herbal shower gels, conditioning shampoos, moisturizing hand soaps, luxurious bubble baths, and more. Complete with a troubleshooting guide and recipes for unique fragrances created by successful soapmakers. 144 pages. Paperback. ISBN 1-58017-243-1.

The Soapmaker's Companion, by Susan Miller Cavitch. The most authoritative guide ever written on making natural, vegetable-based soaps. In addition to basic soapmaking instructions, readers will learn how to use specialty techniques and make transparent, liquid, and imprinted soaps. Includes information on chemistry, ingredients, additives, colorants, and scents. 288 pages. Paperback. ISBN 0-88266-965-6.

Milk-Based Soaps, by Casey Makela. Makela shares her simple technique for making moisturizing milk-based soaps. Covers making classic beauty soaps and specialty soaps, as well as how to turn this hobby into a moneymaker. 112 pages. Paperback. ISBN 0-88266-984-2.

The Natural Soap Book, by Susan Miller Cavitch. An inspiring exploration of the goodness of soap without chemical additives and synthetic ingredients. Step-by-step instructions for creating basic vegetable-based soaps plus suggestions for scenting, coloring, cutting, and wrapping are included. 192 pages. Paperback. ISBN 0-88266-888-9.

The Handmade Soap Book, by Melinda Coss. Using step-by-step instructions and full-color photographs, you can craft a wide variety of bath products from one basic recipe. Create your own unique soaps by experimenting with natural colorings, textures, and scents. 80 pages. Hardcover. ISBN 1-58017-084-6.

The Essential Oils Book, by Colleen K. Dodt. A rich resource on the many applications of aromatherapy and its uses in everyday life including aromas for the home, scents for business environments, and essences for the elderly. 160 pages. Paperback. ISBN 0-88266-913-3.

The Herbal Body Book, by Stephanie Tourles. Learn how to transform common herbs, fruits, and grains into safe, economical, and natural personal care items. Contains over 100 recipes for facial scrubs, hair rinses, shampoos, soaps, cleansing lotions, moisturizers, lip balms, toothpaste, powders, and more! 128 pages. Paperback. ISBN 0-88266-880-3.

The Herbal Home Spa, by Greta Breedlove. These easy-to-make recipes include facial steams, scrubs, masks, and lip balms; massage oils, baths, rubs, and wraps; hand, nail, and foot treatments; and shampoos, dyes, and conditioners. 208 pages. Paperback. ISBN 0-88266-005-6.

These books and other Storey books are available at your bookstore, farm store, garden center, or directly from Storey Books, Schoolhouse Road, Pownal, Vermont 05261, or by calling 800-441-5700. Or visit our Web site at www. storeybooks.com.